THE HEALER WITHIN
The New Medicine of Mind and Body

Steven Locke, M.D., and Douglas Colligan

Foreword by Norman Cousins

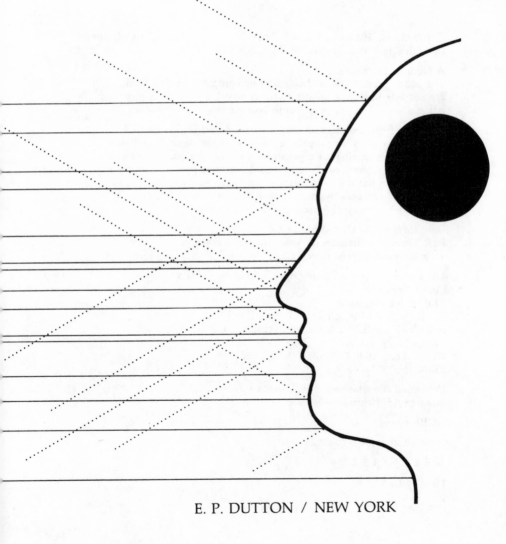

E. P. DUTTON / NEW YORK

To Joanne and Graham, Louise and Deirdre

Published in the United States by
E. P. Dutton, a division of New American Library,
2 Park Avenue, New York, N.Y. 10016.

Library of Congress Cataloging-in-Publication Data
Locke, Steven E.
The healer within.
1. Medicine and psychology. 2. Mind and body.
3. Holistic medicine. 4. Neuropsychiatry. 5. Neuro-
immunology. I. Colligan, Douglas. II. Title.
R726.5.L63   1986   616.08   85-20664
ISBN: 0-525-24283-X

Published simultaneously in Canada by
Fitzhenry & Whiteside Limited, Toronto

COBE

DESIGNED BY MARK O'CONNOR

10 9 8 7 6 5 4 3 2 1

First Edition

THE INSTITUTE OF NOETIC SCIENCES

Astronaut Edgar Mitchell founded this nonprofit membership organization in 1973 to expand knowledge of the nature and potentials of the mind and spirit, and to apply that knowledge to advance health and well-being for humankind and our planet. He chose the word *noetic*—from the Greek "nous", meaning mind, intelligence and understanding; the "noetic sciences", then, are those that *encompass diverse ways of knowing:* the reasoning processes of the intellect, the perceptions of the physical senses, and the intuitive, spiritual, inner ways of knowing.

The Institute funds scientific research; brings top-level scientists and scholars together to share their methods, perspectives and knowledge; and, in publications to its members, discusses new developments in consciousness research.

THE INNER MECHANISMS OF THE HEALING RESPONSE PROGRAM

One of the fundamental goals of the Institute has been to create a scientific understanding of the mind-body relationship. The Institute's Inner Mechanisms Program is devoted to studying *how* the healing response functions. *For example, this Program provided funds to Dr. Steven Locke, co-author of* The Healer Within, *for part of his early research in psychoneuroimmunology—the connection between the mind, emotions and immune system.* The Inner Mechanisms Program asks: What are the innate processes within us that stimulate recovery and natural self-repair? Is there an unknown healing system that promotes remission from normally fatal illnesses? The Institute supports proposals from selected researchers and supports targeted interdisciplinary working conferences on the mechanisms of healing, in areas such as psychoneuroimmunology, energy medicine, spontaneous remission and spiritual healing.

THE EXCEPTIONAL ABILITIES PROGRAM

The Institute seeks to foster a vital, contemporary vision of constructive human potentials—a vision that incorporates all that is known about the farther and higher reaches of human nature. By studying people with outstanding and extraordinary capacities, such as exceptional creativity, physical performance or mental ability, the Institute hopes to learn how individuals can better realize and expand their unique abilities—and, with them, create a world that supports human fulfillment.

THE ALTRUISTIC SPIRIT PROGRAM

In the Altruistic Spirit Program the Institute studies the human capacity for unselfish love and creatively altruistic behavior. The Institute hopes to discover the conditions that foster or suppress creative altruism, and encourage its presence in everyday life.

THE NEW PARADIGMS IN SCIENCE AND SOCIETY PROGRAM

This Program explores the relationship between consciousness—particularly values and beliefs—and global issues, and the premise that *a fundamental change of mind* may be occurring worldwide, for example, in areas such as global peace and common security. In its newest project, "Expanding the Foundations of Science", the Institute is attempting to identify and illuminate what the Institute sees as the changing *foundations* of science—evident in the exciting new developments in physics, biology, the neurosciences, systems theory and other fields. These developments provide startling insights into understanding the basic processes of health and healing, psychology, parapsychology, sociology and international relations. In fact, the Institute believes these changes in the very foundations of science will generate a "global mind change" every bit as sweeping as the dramatic change in worldview accompanying the scientific revolution in the seventeenth century. The New Paradigms Program also explores the role of business in a positive global future.

The Institute's pioneering research and educational programs are financed completely by donations from members and other sources of private support.

Institute members receive a quarterly journal, the *Noetic Sciences Review*, which offers serious discussion of emerging concepts in consciousness research, the mind-body connection and healing, and our changing global reality. Members also receive occasional *Special Reports*, which provide a deeper look into specific issues within these areas; the quarterly *Noetic Sciences Bulletin*, with reports on continuing Institute projects, member activities, and upcoming conferences and lectures; and *An Intelligent Guide*, a comprehensive catalog of the many books, audiotapes and videotapes in this field, which are available to members at a discount.

The Institute of Noetic Sciences
475 Gate Five Road, Suite 300
Sausalito, California 94965-0909
(415) 331-5650

Contents

CONTENTS

vi

Acknowledgments

WE WOULD LIKE to express our appreciation to the individuals and organizations whose assistance and support were invaluable. For editorial assistance to Bennett Simon, Linda J. Kraus, Linda Shirer, and Theodore Melnechuk. For research to Joanne Callahan Locke, Elizabeth R. Power, and Linda N. Cabot as well as Barbara Ford, Ruth Borgman, and Leah Wallach. For other editorial assistance, our gratitude goes to Graham S. Bengen for his help in photocopying, to Nancy Lucas for her speedy and accurate tape transcription, and to Murray Cox for his stamina in typing, retyping, and retyping yet again.

Of immeasurable value for their enthusiasm and encouragement are Leonore Savage, M. Barry Flint, and Harris Dienstfrey of the Institute for the Advancement of Health, and Joan and Myrin Borysenko, valued friends and colleagues. This work was supported in part by a grant from the Institute of Noetic Sciences, Sausalito, California. The assistance and encouragement of Brendan O'Regan of the Institute is especially appreciated.

Finally, a personal note of thanks to our agent Barbara Lowenstein for setting it all in motion, to Paul De Angelis and Caroline Press for their conscientious and professional work on an immensely complex topic, to Susan Thornton for her superb copy editing, and to our families whose patience and generosity with their own time went beyond the call of duty.

Foreword

THE LATE Franz Ingelfinger, in an article for *The New England Journal of Medicine,* of which he was editor, wrote that 85 percent of the illnesses physicians are called upon to treat are self-limiting. That is, without any help, the human body is able in most cases to prescribe for itself. It does so because of a healing system that is no less real than the circulatory system, the digestive system, the nervous system, or any of the other systems that define human beings and enable them to function.

We are here confronted, however, with one of the great paradoxes of medical science. Less is known and taught about the healing system than about any of the other internal forces that govern human existence. Eight years ago, when I first came into the medical community, I tried to find out as much as I could about the way the body heals itself—whether with respect to a cut finger or inflammation of the joints or stomach disorders or a cold or a major disease —and kept running into a blank wall. I looked for "healing system" in the indices of medical textbooks and found nothing. I turned to the standard medical dictionaries and saw no entry for "healing system," though I found entries for all the other major systems. I looked in the standard manuals—such as Merck's—with the same lack of success. I consulted the curriculum catalogues of medical schools and found listings for anatomy, physiology, endocrinology, pathology, psychology, immunology, physics, biophysics, and chemistry, but, again, nothing on the way the total organism is equipped to recover from abnormalities and illnesses.

My colleagues at the medical school told me that the various components included in healing were taught under separate rubrics. There was a great deal, for example, on the immune system—or the way different categories of cells act singly and in combination to protect the body against disease as well as to try to overcome it. But the fact that the healing system was not taught as a fully integrated entity seemed strange to me. The view that Steven Locke and Douglas Colligan bring into focus reveals a grand potentiation and orchestration of all the body's systems in enabling human beings to meet a serious challenge. Most of all, the book shows how mind and body interact—how the emotions affect biology, how the nervous system, the endocrine system, and the immune system function in relation to each other. In so doing, the authors not only fill a long-felt need but also join the growing group of medical pioneers who are opening up new vistas in understanding how the human body repairs itself.

Not so long ago, the term *psychosomatic medicine* was adequate to describe or encompass the effect of mind on body or body on mind. In recent years, however, enlarged understanding of the way the body's systems interact has led to new and perhaps more sophisticated terms such as *psychoneuroimmunology* and *psychobiology*. A new science is emerging, and Dr. Locke is among its main figures.

As might be expected, any new thrust in science is apt to produce some misinterpretation and even contention. One of the prime tenets of the new work is that psychological factors can play a part in causing disease—all the way from colds to cancer. It is inevitable perhaps that this thesis would be wrongly interpreted in some circles. Indeed, a debate erupted over an article in *The New England Journal of Medicine* for June 13, 1985, titled, "Psychosocial

Correlates of Survival in Advanced Malignant Disease?" Primary author of the article was Dr. Barrie Cassileth of the University of Pennsylvania Cancer Center in Philadelphia. The authors reported on a study of 359 persons with severe malignancies. The death rate was 75 percent. The conclusion of the study was that, in cases of high-risk advanced cancer, only the inherent biology of the disease determined the outcome, and that psychological, emotional, or other factors were largely irrelevant in treatment.

Dr. Cassileth's article led to reports in the popular press, especially in the news magazines, that it had been finally and "certifiably" demonstrated that positive emotions, such as hope, will to live, faith, laughter and good spirits, purpose and determination, had little to do with health and were not useful in combatting disease. There was a reference to old-wives' tales. Yet a careful reading of Dr. Cassileth's article supported no such interpretations. She was writing about certain kinds of malignancies for which, at present, neither medical nor psychological treatment offers sufficient promise. But *high-risk, advanced cancer* accounts for only a tiny fraction—less than 4 percent—of all illnesses in the United States. Her study was never intended to apply to the 96 percent of all illnesses in which the emotions—negative or positive—have some degree of involvement. And even in advanced malignancies, psychological or psychosocial factors have a great deal to do with a patient's quality of life.

Dr. Cassileth was disturbed over the interpretations given her article and over the fact that it was being used to refute my own work at the UCLA School of Medicine. Her telephone call led to a decision to issue a joint statement in which the following points were made:

1. Emotions and health are closely related;
2. Probably numerous emotional and physical factors influence health and disease;
3. Positive attitudes affect the quality of life even where they cannot influence the physical outcome of disease;
4. Panic, not uncommon when cancer is diagnosed, is, in itself, destructive and can interfere with effective treatment.

All these points receive detailed exposition in the present volume, which, to my mind, is the most explicit and complete account of the nature of the human healing system and, more particularly, of the scientific verification for the way emotions and attitudes—negative or positive—can affect health and the treatment of disease. Dr. Locke's account is not theoretical but draws upon the results of experiments and research reports throughout the world to show how the mind can affect the body, and vice versa. These findings have led to the concept of the brain as an apothecary capable of filling a wide array of prescriptions for the body, including pain-killers.

In this connection, the authors refer to the experiences of thousands of persons who have walked across hot embers, in so-called firewalks, without injury. Having witnessed some of these fire-walks, I can attest to the fact that everyday individuals can, without pain or injury, actually walk across a bed of hot ashes. I would not, however, advise anyone to attempt a homemade firewalk in an attempt to replicate the experience. While it is undoubtedly true that psychological factors play a part in enabling individuals to sustain pain, these factors are operative only up to a certain point. Emotions or attitudes are not absolutes. They provide an impressive degree of protection for a limited amount of time, varying with certain circumstances and the individual involved.

There is no question about the fact that the ashes in the fire-walk are hot, nor is there any question about the fact that the intense emotional preparation prior to the firewalk—preparation running into several hours and often leading to a state of quasihys-teria also observable at Holy Roller excitations—figures in the final result. But there are limits, which accounts for the fact that some individuals do experience pain, burning, and blisters. I didn't fire-walk with the others. I had no intention of being anything other than an observer. I didn't understand the phenomenon and was certain I would be blistered. My education made me conscious of the physical laws of cause and effect; i.e., if a flame is put to flesh, the flesh would burn. If a crowbar comes down on a human arm with sufficient force, the bone in the arm will break.

Natural laws have to be respected. But I also realized that while my doubts would probably predispose me to blistering, the pro-found confidence of others would predispose them to a more salu-tary result. A friend of mine who is a psychiatrist had similar mis-givings but decided to go across the hot ashes just the same; he was blistered.

What to me was most fascinating about the firewalks is not the fact that most individuals come through it without burns or blisters but that some of them don't. What accounts for the difference? In my own limited experience as observer, I find it significant that those who are blistered are generally highly educated persons who are skeptical of the experience to begin with. For example, my psychiatrist friend participated in the "warm-up" exercises, which lasted about three hours and which were designed to put the group, numbering more than a hundred persons, into a state of blazing confidence and determination—a feeling that nothing was beyond their reach. The leader or guru was Tony Robbins, a tall, charismatic young man. He led the group through a series of emotional exercises similar to collective hypnosis. The purpose seemed to me to be twofold: first, to transfer the group's will to its leader, enabling him to cause the group to laugh or weep or exult at his command; second, to enable the members of the group to experience a sense of personal power unlike anything they had known before. When the leader saw that the people were ready, he told them the firewalk would be like cool moss beneath their feet. In fact, they would chant the words "cool moss" while they walked across the firewalk.

While the group was being indoctrinated, I went outside to inspect the setting. Attendants had built a fire on the ground in an area approximately four feet wide and ten feet long. The distance could be traversed in three or four steps. Logs, not coal, were burned. I noticed that the attendants had turned a water hose on the ground fore and aft of the "firebox." How important moist feet were to the desired result I have no way of knowing. Another equivocal factor was that the residue of the fire was not hot coals, as was the general impression, but the thick and soft ash produced by wood. This is not to say that the ash didn't generate substantial heat. I felt uncomfortably hot just standing a few feet from the ash. But it must be emphasized, nevertheless, that the people didn't walk on hot coals.

When the participants emerged from their indoor session, many of them seemed transported. Just before each person started across the firewalk, Tony Robbins scrutinized their eyes to make certain they were ready. He reminded them to chant "cool moss," then would tap them on the back and release them for the three or four steps across the hot ashes.

I observed my psychiatrist friend as he waited his turn. It

appeared to me that he was not as wide-eyed and emotionally supercharged as were most of the others. When he stepped forward, Robbins peered into his eyes, tapped him on the back, and sent him across the ashes. My friend stomped forward, chanting "cool moss," and completed the journey in three steps. He seemed to feel nothing at the time, he said, but three or four seconds later he became aware that he had burned himself and had to be treated. The burns were not serious and didn't require hospitalization or anything like that; but they were more than merely uncomfortable. Clearly, his experience was unlike that of most of the others. This fact to me was perhaps more significant than the fact that most of the others experienced no burns at all. For what it said to me was that, despite the ash from wood rather than coals, and despite the moistening of the feet just before and after the firewalk, there *was* some risk of getting at least minor burns. Was it possible that my friend the psychiatrist, who had admitted to me that he had been skeptical about the entire procedure all along but was eager to submit himself to the experiment in order to learn more about it, never reached the state of emotional frenzy or hypnosis that was essential to the enterprise?

I was able to draw no clear-cut conclusions from the episode. It was obvious to me that some aspects of the firewalk were not as advertised. Ash from wood cools off very rapidly. In this case it was thick enough to offer some measure of protection from the hot embers below—exactly how much protection, I had no way of knowing. Next, how essential were moist soles to the desired result? (When I asked about the wet ground, I was told that it was necessary to prevent the spread of fire. The reply was not entirely satisfactory since it would have been possible for the participants to have had a moist-free narrow path leading onto and away from the "firewalk.") When I asked why the walk was only three or four steps, I was told that firewalks up to and over twenty feet had been successfully conducted.

Taking everything into account, I felt that the test was equivocal, that the group hypnosis or transport had imparted some degree of protection but not enough to set aside the natural laws that would have unquestionably come into play with ash from hot coals and with unmoistened feet, but that the degree of belief had some bearing on the extent to which even the limited risk could be successfully sustained. The fact that my friend had fallen short seemed to indicate the existence of an individual threshold. An equation was apparently at work in which the factors involved were degrees of heat, degrees of protection, and degrees of belief.

Similar examples of the power of belief to create biochemical or physiological change are cited in this book. The significance of such phenomena, of course, is represented by their relevance in health and healing. If what one thinks can affect one's internal organs and tissues under ordinary circumstances, how can mental processes be put to use under circumstances of need or challenge? It is with respect to questions such as these that this book is of special value.

I had an opportunity to observe the interplay of attitudes, emotions, and physiology in a group of seriously ill persons known as the Wellness Community in Santa Monica, California. The group had been organized by Harold Benjamin, a public-spirited local citizen who believed deeply in the importance of environmental factors in the treatment of cancer. He provided a "community center" for cancer patients, where they could come together for mutual emotional support. These emotional needs were no less real than their physical needs.

After several years of existence, the Wellness Community has one clearly documented attribute: its members, with few exceptions, have outlived the predictions of their physicians. I met with the group in an effort to seek information on this development. Did the individual members have any theories about their longevity? Could they identify any single event or turning point that led to their improved prospects?

One woman volunteered a reply. She was in her upper seventies but was uncommonly beautiful. This was the way Grace Kelly might have looked, I thought, if she had lived to that age. The woman had a clear idea, she said, of when the turning point for the better occurred. It was at her physician's office, at the very beginning. "Mrs. A.," he had said, "we have completed our examination and I am making an unequivocal diagnosis of cancer. It is terminal and I give you four to six months."

Mrs. A. said she looked her physician squarely in the eyes and said: "Go f--- yourself."

Nothing could be more incongruous than hearing this gracious, distinguished lady using such explicit language, but she had a point to make—and the other patients cheered. Most of them had had similar experiences. They did not deny the diagnosis. What they denied was the verdict that went with it; and they protested the arrogance of anyone who would presume to "give" anyone a certain number of months to live.

I asked Mrs. A. how long ago the encounter with the physician had occurred. She said almost six and a half years.

When I went around the room, I discovered that most of the patients had lived at least three years beyond the forecasts of their physicians. Why should determination and a blazing will to live make such a difference? New research on the interaction between the mind, the endocrine system, and the immune system promises to furnish answers to these questions and, in so doing, tell us more than we have ever known before about the uniqueness of human life. Steven Locke is one of the leading pioneers in this field. His book enables the reader to join him on one of history's most exciting scientific journeys.

—Norman Cousins

CHAPTER ONE

The Reunion
of Mind
and Body

ANCIENT CHINESE MEDICAL texts discuss the concept of *Fu-zheng*, the natural enhancement of a person's mechanisms for fighting disease. Following are three stories of Fu-zheng in action. The first occurs at what many might consider to be an improbable place, Harvard University.

THE HEALER AND THE PSYCHOLOGIST

A few years ago in a little-noted experiment, Harvard psychologist David McClelland tried out his own Fu-zheng experiment, using as his research tools a telephone, the common cold, some cooperative undergraduates, and a healer. It is important to understand who

1

David McClelland is. He is one of the most honored and influential professionals in the field of motivational psychology. His teaching has shaped the careers of generations of the most innovative and articulate psychologists around. (He is also the man who hired, and fired, LSD guru Timothy Leary.) He is a self-described maverick who mildly startled a group of his colleagues by telling them that he goes to a psychic healer, often with beneficial results.

As part of his fascination with the process of healing, he asked a group of Harvard students to participate in a Fu-zheng experiment with his healer. Anyone who felt he was getting a cold was to call a certain number. Within twenty-four hours of the phone call, each was taken to the healer. To each student, the healer either declared (entirely at whim), "You're healed" or suggested healing by saying to another student, "You heal him. I give my power to you."

To measure the success rate of the healer, McClelland listed thirty-two symptoms indicating the severity or weakness of the cold before and after the visit. He also measured levels of an antibody, immunoglobulin A (IgA), in their saliva. (IgA is in protective secretions that help the immune system to resist upper respiratory illnesses—colds, flu, sinus problems.) After the healing ritual, nine of the thirteen students who had felt their colds abate also had higher levels of IgA.

One result of this experiment, McClelland says, was that it irritated the nonpsychic healers (the doctors) at the Harvard University Health Service. "The doctors had their noses put a little out of joint by this," he admits. "They said, 'Hell, just take them [the students with colds] to the health services at Harvard, tell them they're better, and they'll *get* better.'"

So, McClelland did. At random half of the undergraduates having the classic symptoms of a cold went to the University Health Service, and half to his healer. Again, none of the students touched by the healer developed a cold; all of those who went to the clinic developed severe colds.

CANCER "CURES," CANCER CURSES

Probably no doctor alive has not seen or heard of a patient's recovery from a disease that defied conventional medical explanations.

2

Most are noted momentarily and quickly forgotten, another medical oddity. But one physician, Bruno Klopfer, documented a spectacularly complex case that lives on in the folklore of medicine.[1]

His story involved a patient named Mr. Wright who had cancer of the lymph nodes. The standard treatments were tried and failed. It soon became obvious to the doctor and the hospital staff treating him that Mr. Wright had little time left. His body was bloated with tumors, some the size of oranges. Every day one or two quarts of a milky fluid was drained from his chest. With little else to offer, the hospital staff spent most of their time trying to make Wright as comfortable as possible in preparation for his inevitable death.

But Wright was not ready to die. He had heard about a new, experimental cancer drug, Krebiozen, and wanted to try it. By luck the clinic where the doctor worked was selected to test the drug. Wright asked to be included in the trial, but his physician refused his request, on the grounds that the drug supply was limited and was to be used only on patients who had resisted conventional therapies and had at least a few months of life remaining. Wright was expected to last no more than two weeks. But Wright pleaded for the drug. Finally, the doctor relented, mostly out of pity, and included him in the thrice-weekly injection schedule. He gave Wright the first injection on a Friday and went home.

On Monday he arrived at the hospital, half expecting to find Wright had died or was dying. He found instead that the gasping, moribund man he had left in a hospital bed Friday was now walking around, talking pleasantly with the other patients and with the nurses. His tumors had shrunk to half their original size, and this once-dying man now seemed only slightly ill. His improvement was, in the physician's words, "brilliant." Within ten days of his first Krebiozen injection, Wright was out of his bed and out of the hospital. He was, so far as his doctors could tell, disease free.

Soon afterward new reports about Krebiozen began to appear in the press, and the news was the same: Krebiozen was ineffectual. Coincident with these reports, Wright had a relapse after enjoying two months of relatively good health and was readmitted to the hospital.

Since more than biochemistry was obviously at work inside Wright, the doctor decided to double-check this suspicious drug, this time using Wright as a *control* patient in the study, someone who received a harmless substitute for the drug. "This scheme could not

3

harm him in any way, I felt sure," he told Klopfer, "and anyway there was nothing I knew that could help him."

The physician told Wright that he would receive a double-strength dosage of a new, improved type of Krebiozen. To build up a little anticipation and suspense, the doctor delayed giving Wright the drug. With elaborate medical ceremony, he approached his patient's bed and carefully injected him with the "new" Krebiozen.

As before, within days of the injections, Wright's tumors shrank away and the fluid in his chest disappeared. The hospital staff were stunned by Wright's improvement, especially since he had received only injections of sterile water. Wright again left the hospital and resumed a life that was symptom-free for the following two months.

That second respite ended when a story appeared in the newspaper with an important announcement from the American Medical Association: "Nationwide tests show Krebiozen to be a worthless drug in treatment of cancer." A few days later Mr. Wright appeared at the hospital, riddled with tumors. The doctor described his patient's state of mind and its final result: "His faith was now gone, his last hope vanished, and he succumbed in less than two days."

By contrast, a team of Japanese doctors at Kyushu University's School of Medicine have recorded the account of Mr. H. as part of their study of spontaneous regression of cancer, cases of people whose disease receded for no apparent reason.[2] In one instance a sixty-five-year-old man, a devout member of the Shinto sect, complained to his doctor of nosebleeds. The medical exam detected the underlying problem as cancer of the jaw. Surgeons located the growth and removed it. A few months later the man returned to the physician, this time complaining of severe laryngitis. His sore throat turned out to be cancer of a vocal cord. The doctor recommended surgery. The patient would not allow it. He was a dedicated church leader who preached regularly. He preferred to continue to preach with the cancer in his throat rather than have it cut out and to risk losing his voice entirely. Not only did he refuse surgery, but he would not agree to radiation therapy or to chemotherapy. "This is God's will," he said of his cancer diagnosis, "and I have no complaint about it. Whatever should happen will just happen." A few days later, Mr. H. visited his religious leader, who told him, "You are an invaluable asset for our church." Touched by the compliment, Mr. H. returned home, determined to refuse treatment and to keep preaching as long as his voice held out.

A short time later he was standing before his congregation and, in a hoarse, strained voice, managed to deliver a brief sermon, just a few minutes long. Months later, six months after his diagnosis, he was still speaking publicly. By then his sermons were thirty minutes long, and the weakness and hoarseness in his voice had disappeared.

Years later, an amazed doctor, after peering into Mr. H.'s throat, reported: "This patient seemed to be drastically cured. When I looked into his throat . . . the tumor was gone." Thirteen years after his diagnosis, Mr. H. died at age seventy-eight, of complications from a back injury.

DR. KIRKPATRICK AND THE WITCH

During the late 1970s Dr. Richard Kirkpatrick, a Longview, Washington, physician, had a twenty-eight-year-old Filipino woman patient, who complained that she felt weak. Routine medical tests showed the woman was suffering from *systemic lupus erythematosus*, a disease in which the body's immune system attacks its own body's tissue: heart, lung, kidneys. Lupus has no cure, but it can be treated. It can also go into remission, disappearing for years as suddenly as it appeared.

Kirkpatrick prescribed standard drugs. None had much effect. More complications appeared. Other drugs and a kidney biopsy were prescribed. This time the woman balked at the treatment and left town. She flew back to the remote village in the Philippines where she was born. There she consulted her local witch doctor. He explained to her why she had the disease: An old boyfriend had put a curse on her. In a special ceremony he removed the curse and told her to go back to the United States, but to refuse additional tests and medicine.

Three weeks later she returned to Washington, by all medical measures completely recovered. Because lupus is a very labile disease, her remission was not surprising. The speed with which she recovered, not only from the disease but also from the side effects of some of the potent drugs she had taken, however, defied medical explanation. Kirkpatrick was so impressed with the case that he described it in the *Journal of the American Medical Association (JAMA)*

5

under the title "Witchcraft and Lupus Erythematosus."[3] (Two and a half years later a small note appeared in *JAMA*. For the first time since her visit to the witch doctor, the woman returned to Kirkpatrick with another problem, a small cyst. This time she let him take a blood test. There was still no sign of the disease.)

Stories of mysterious recoveries have existed as long as medicine has. In dealing with these anomalies, all that doctors could do was to give them Latinate names—the placebo effect, remission, psychogenic disease—and move on to what they could handle more easily. The level of medical technology borders on the miraculous sometimes. As a matter of medical routine doctors can, with a simple injection, make a person immune to some of the deadliest diseases on the planet. Smallpox, for example, is an extinct disease now. In the operating room surgeons can deliberately take individuals to the brink of death, even stop the heart, and restore them again. To a doctor practicing at the turn of the century, half of what is now medically routine would seem miraculous.

Yet writing on the future of medical schools, Derek Bok, president of Harvard University, declared that a new way of training doctors must be devised. He said that the modern doctor is in danger of being buried by information and overwhelmed by technology. Medical students today attend endless lectures during which they are bombarded by volumes of scientific information. Yet some of what they remember may be of marginal use in years to come. One survey found that four out of ten doctors admitted they could no longer keep pace with developments in their own fields.

The great frustration is that there remain arenas of medicine that technology cannot reach. Harvard Medical School cardiologist Dr. Herbert Benson, the discoverer of the relaxation response, says that the arsenal of techniques and medicines at doctors' disposal allow them to cure only about one-fourth of the illnesses that plague humankind. The rest are either incurable or self-limiting; that is, somehow or another they heal themselves.

Doctors have long been aware of an element to healing that does not appear in a microscope or yield its secrets to a battery of blood tests. Some element in the mind of the patient makes an important difference in the body's reaction to illness, something as ephemeral as an attitude or feeling that could leave its mark on the body.

For many doctors the notion that emotions can influence body processes is folklore. This attitude has not always prevailed. Hippocrates suggested that there were *natural* as well as divine causes for disease, and that these causes were discernible by the use of reason. He also thought that being healthy was evidence that an individual had achieved a state of harmony, both within himself and within his environment. In this view, staying healthy is largely a matter of recognizing this equilibrium and respecting it by living according to natural laws. Further, he believed that whatever happens in the mind affects what happens in the body.

Part of Hippocrates' medical theory was his concept of health as maintaining a balance of four vital bodily fluids, or humours: blood, yellow bile, black bile, and phlegm. According to some ancient practitioners, blood came from the heart, yellow bile from the liver, black bile from the spleen, and phlegm from the brain. These fluids influenced the body and the brain. Ideally harmony prevailed among these humours, but where one dominated a personality, a characteristic state of mind accompanied it. That concept has shaped our vocabulary today. When we talk of a *phlegmatic* individual or feeling *sanguine* about a subject or describe someone as *bilious,* we pay homage to this ancient theory.

Hippocrates and others believed that the climate where a person lived determined the characteristic interrelationship of these humours. Specifically, Hippocrates noted in his famous treatise on the subject that the combined influence of "air, water, and places" directly influenced the humours inside a person, so that a person's humours, and therefore his health, were affected by his environment. Today this theory sounds primitive, but the basic idea behind the humoral theory has proved amazingly durable.

These ancient medical truths faded from consciousness for a while, eclipsed by changes in the philosophy and technology of medicine. Philosophically, the single most powerful influence for change was the seventeenth-century French philosopher René Descartes. He declared that individuals had two distinct components: the ethereal abstraction we call the *mind* and the concrete body. The study of each required a different methodology. The key to studying the mind was self-reflection and dialogue with others. The key to studying the body was to analyze it as a masterwork of biomechanics. And in Descartes's time, this was virgin territory for scientific exploration.

Descartes even bequeathed to medical science a scientific method for researchers to employ in their explorations. To learn about the complex, he said, study the simple. Learn about a germ and you eventually know something about the disease associated with it.

This new *reductionist method,* as it came to be known, was the dominant concept of medicine in the centuries that followed. In its support another medical theory came to prominence, again in France. It was known as the *theory of specific etiology,* the idea that every disease or infection is caused by an identifiable microorganism. The theory received strong support from research done by Robert Koch, a Prussian medical officer and scientific dilettante fascinated by bacteria. By today's standards, when we award researchers a Nobel prize and elevate them to the pantheon of great scientists for a single discovery, Koch's accomplishments were breathtaking. He solved the mystery of the life cycle of the deadly livestock disease anthrax, isolated the tubercule bacillus, and later developed a vaccine for diphtheria.

A contemporary of Koch's, Louis Pasteur, took the discovery a step further by finding a cure for anthrax. Historians write of Pasteur's standing in a field littered with the bodies of sheep, acknowledging the applause of a small crowd of scientists. He had just demonstrated the possibility of protecting animals against anthrax by exposing some of them to a weakened version of the deadly disease. Once acquainted with the disease, the animals' immune system, the natural system of self-defense, was able to withstand a full dose of the virulent killer. Those not inoculated died within a few days.

He extended his interest to humans and made medical history by injecting a boy, bitten by a rabid dog, with a series of weak solutions of rabies. The experiment saved the boy's life, demonstrated a treatment for rabies, and showed that the principle of specific etiology was valid and had important medical implications. The success of the rabies experiment gave Pasteur and others the courage to attempt immunization against other diseases.

Listening to the gospel of specific etiology, researchers mobilized their talents and their laboratories. Barely a year went by without some stunning scientific breakthrough. Diseases that had been the scourge of humankind were dropping before one magic bullet after another. In 1906 researchers used Koch's discovery of the tuberculin bacillus to develop a vaccine for the disease. In 1911 researchers developed a special arsenic compound, Salvarsan, that effectively treated many forms of syphilis. In the 1920s insulin was isolated, and insulin injections were extending the lifetimes of diabetic patients. In the 1930s sulfa drugs appeared and, with them, cures for bacterial pneumonia, meningitis, gonorrhea, and urinary tract infections. By the 1940s the sulfa drugs were largely replaced by even more potent drugs, the antibiotics, made possible by the discovery of penicillin. It seemed that there was no disease that medical science could not handle.

For most of the history of modern medicine this biomedical approach has dominated the philosophy of science for the best of all reasons: it worked. Small wonder that scientist-author René Dubos called the doctrine of specific etiology "the most powerful single force in the development of medicine during the past century."[4]

THE LOST ART OF HEALING

As the science of healing improved, the art experienced traumatic changes. The biomedical approach tended to put some distance between doctor and patient, partly because the disease as much as the patient dominated the doctor's attention. Medical historians generally agree that one of the first pieces of technology that set into motion the depersonalizing process in medicine appeared in 1819. Then a French physician, René Laennec, wrote a tremendously valuable book describing the technique of *auscultation,* the science of making diagnoses by listening to internal sounds of the human body. It gave the doctor a whole new way of collecting information about the patient's heart, lungs, and belly with the aid of Laennec's new piece of medical hardware, the stethoscope.

This marvelous tool allowed doctors to make more accurate and informative examinations of the internal organs of their patients. It also transformed the ritual of the physical examination forever. As physician-author Lewis Thomas points out in *The Youngest Science,* it eliminated the old practice of pressing one's ear to the patient's chest. The stethoscope replaced this gesture with something more informative, but less intimate. It eliminated the soothing effect of human touch, which Thomas describes as "the oldest and most effective act of doctors."[5]

He goes on to explain:

Touching with the naked ear was one of the great advances in the history of medicine. Once it was learned that the heart and lungs made sounds of their own, and that the sounds were sometimes useful for diagnosis, physicians placed an ear over the heart, and over areas on the front and back of the chest, and listened. It is hard to imagine a friendlier human gesture, a more intimate signal of personal concern and affection, than the close-bowed head affixed to the skin.

By the mid-1800s other diagnostic instruments joined the stethoscope in the doctor's bag: the ophthalmoscope (for examining eyes), the laryngoscope (for the throat), and the otoscope (for the ears).

Clinical tests and technologies used for diagnosis further reinforced the image of patient as an object of study. By the turn of the century, doctors had tests for tuberculosis, diphtheria, typhoid, cholera, and syphilis. Soon after came the X ray, the electrocardiogram, the electroencephalogram, and blood tests. The patient became less and less a fellow human with an illness and more and more an amalgam of medical data. And the result, some feel, is that today we have ceased to be patients and have become specimens.

It is sometimes forgotten that as technology came to play more and more of a dominant role in the practice of medicine, other forces, which would gradually revive interest in the mind and its influence on the health of the body, were at work. One person who played a pivotal role in reevaluating the significance of the mind as an element in health and disease was a young Viennese neurologist, Sigmund Freud. In the 1880s Freud had traveled to Paris, where he spent months attending the lectures of a brilliant nineteenth-century French neurologist, Jean-Martin Charcot. Although he is all but forgotten today, Charcot was known as the "Napoleon of neurosis." His studies of the human mind dominated that field of study.

When Freud was in Paris, Charcot was the head of the Salpetrière, a famous Parisian hospital for the poor that he had turned into one of the greatest research hospitals in the world. There Charcot put on his famous Friday-morning lectures, which were pure theater. His talks were immensely popular; the lecture hall was usually filled with an expectant crowd long before Charcot appeared.

A favorite demonstration of Charcot's was to summon to the front of the lecture hall a mental patient suffering from hysterical paralysis. Under hypnosis the patient would stand and walk at Charcot's bidding. When taken out of the trance, the same person would crumple to the ground, crippled once again. His public demonstrations showed dramatically the way that a state of mind could affect the body and could even be manipulated. Charcot's fascination with the healing powers of the mind became a lifelong preoccupation. In the latter part of his life, he examined patients who had been miraculously cured after a visit to Lourdes.

Freud undoubtedly witnessed some of Charcot's hypnosis "cures" of paralyzed patients and in time himself would theorize that emotions not expressed in words or actions would find expression in some sort of physical ailment. This was the germ of his concept of *conversion hysteria.* Essentially, Freud held that chronic emotional problems could develop into physical ones. (The word *Hysteria* is from the Greek word for "uterus"; it had been universally assumed that only women suffered from conversion disorders, real ailments with no discernible physical cause.) Charcot rediscovered and reasserted the idea that the phenomenon could affect men as well (an idea dating to the time of Galen eighteen hundred years ago), when he documented a case of hysteria in a German grenadier.

Freud took Charcot's work a little further, suggesting that the physical symptoms of hysteria were connected to some past experience. In situations in which one person might cry, rage, or otherwise express some emotional reaction to a traumatic event, the hysteric, Freud suggested, might find the experience too painful to contemplate, relegating the memory to the unconscious. Later that emotional reaction might return in the form of some physical problem.

In time, specialists in all fields began to notice something they called *organ neurosis,* disturbances of the internal organs. Terms such as *gastric, intestinal,* and *cardiac neurosis* entered the medical lexicon to describe emotionally triggered problems of the stomach, bowels, and heart.

Others believed that illness was sometimes more than the simple cause and effect, germ-attacks-body scenario. One of the first to suggest this interpretation was Claude Bernard, a great nineteenth-century French physiologist, an expert in the workings of

11

the body. Bernard made several breakthrough discoveries: that the liver stores blood sugar and releases it as the body needs it; that pancreatic fluid helps to digest food; that the nervous system helps regulate the flow of blood in the body.

Bernard was also a philosopher of medicine. He talked of the *milieu interieur* of the body, the concept that the body was always working to maintain a delicate balance in its chemistry and the functioning of its many parts. When this balance was disturbed, sickness and death could result.

Another physiologist fascinated with a holistic view of the body was Dr. Walter Cannon, a physiologist at Harvard Medical School in the 1930s and 1940s. Building on Bernard's insights, he tried to discover the elements that kept this internal environment harmonious. The body, he concluded, enjoyed a state of self-maintaining health, which Cannon called *homeostasis.* This acts as a kind of bodily gyroscope, keeping the internal environment stable.

One system vital to homeostasis is the immune system. This is the body's built-in biochemical defense against disease and infection. Healers have known about it for centuries and learned to use it. As long as two thousand years ago, Chinese doctors knew it could be directed and had a crude system of vaccination called *variolation.* They injected live smallpox organisms into individuals. (Those who didn't die from the procedure were immunized for life.) Twentieth-century shamans had their own, more sophisticated biochemical weapons—vaccines and sulfa drugs—to complement the immune system's abilities.

Over time, scientists made other discoveries. They learned that if immune cells were released in a test tube full of enemy microbes, the cells would dispatch the microbes with the same efficiency as in the body. This led immunologists to conclude that the immune system was unique among the bodily systems because it functioned autonomously.

During the first half of this century, researchers also learned that the immune system could tell which cells belonged to its own body and which were foreign; that it had a biochemical memory that helped it recognize and destroy foreign cells; that it was capable of dispatching as many as ten million different microbial enemies.

But it was not until the late 1950s that scientists began to learn in finer detail how the immune system did what it did. Around that time a British biochemist named Rodney Porter and an American immunologist, Gerald Edelman, determined the precise molecular structure of an antibody, the germ-fighting component of the immune system. This won them a Nobel prize and ushered in the era of a new immunology, one that has given us the most detailed view in history of this homeostatic system.

But as long ago as 1935, Walter Cannon said that homeostasis was more than the nervous system and biochemicals working in harmony with one another. He suggested the normal experiences of life—the onset of puberty and the agony of adolescence, fatigue, hard work, everyday worry—all made a physical impression on the body. "Indeed," Cannon observed, "the whole gamut of human diseases might be studied from this point of view."

While Cannon was studying the process through which the body regulated itself, psychoanalytic theory, an outgrowth of Freud's work, was finding applications for various physical ailments. One of the first to see its potential was Chicago psychiatrist Dr. Franz Alexander. In 1939, Alexander made what was for that time the outlandish statement that "many chronic disturbances are not caused by external, mechanical, chemical factors or by microorganisms, but by the continuous functional stress arising during the everyday life of the organism in its struggle for existence."[6] His ideas were to evolve into the new discipline of *psychosomatic medicine,* which revived the ancient belief in the mind as an important component in physical health.

According to Alexander, several developments had set the stage for this new medicine. One was Cannon's discovery that many functions of the body were controlled by a central nervous system. Another was the discovery of ductless glands such as the adrenal and pituitary glands, which empty their powerful secretions into the bloodstream. Cannon also pointed out that the entire nervous system is in turn controlled by a central regulatory agency "which in human beings we call the personality."[7]

Out of his work came the psychoanalytic approach to medicine, examining the events in the person's mind, as well as the body. That technique placed the mind-body relationship under a Freudian microscope. By the 1950s, psychosomaticists had a list of seven psychosomatic ailments: peptic ulcers, ulcerative colitis, hypertension, hyperthyroidism, rheumatoid arthritis, neurodermatitis, and asthma, diseases considered to have a potent psychological as well as a physical component. (The idea of a separate category of psy-

13

chosomatic diseases generated much excitement and controversy, which continue to this day. Followers of Alexander were not able to demonstrate that continual stress was the cause of any given disease. And specific studies of the psychosomatic seven showed them to be much more complicated than originally thought. No single cause could explain them all.)

As psychosomaticists were piling up their evidence about the role of the mind in disease, a brilliant Austro-Hungarian organic chemist named Hans Selye was hard at work at McGill University in Montreal, putting together his major contributions to medical science: the discovery and naming of the phenomenon he called "stress," to which Franz Alexander alluded, and the analysis of its medical and psychological effects. After his laboratory rats received a series of shocks or injections, their bodies registered the effect. Although to all appearances the stressed rats suffered little physical harm, Selye's autopsies found physical damage, withered and spent glands, in the wake of the pressures on the animals.[8]

By the 1960s other evidence had accumulated showing the effects of the mind on the body. At the Rockefeller University in New York, psychologist Dr. Neal Miller believed that it would be possible to apply Cannon's discovery about the nervous system's control over the body. Miller decided to try conditioned learning techniques to direct functions once considered involuntary. He managed to train a group of rats to raise or lower their heart rate or blood pressure on command by sending a pulse of electricity to the "pleasure centers" of their brains. In time the rats became so skilled that they could relax or contract specific muscles of their intestines and even control the flow of blood to one or both of their ears. In one swoop those mysterious feats of the yogis—raising the temperature of one hand or racing or slowing the beat of their hearts —did not seem so mysterious.

In the meantime in Boston, Dr. Herbert Benson, a respected cardiologist at Harvard Medical School, was studying the relationship between stress and hypertension. In stressful situations the body undergoes a variety of changes: rise in blood pressure and pulse, and faster breathing. Benson reasoned that if stress could turn on this reaction, some other factor might be able to turn it off.

During the early 1970s Benson had been studying experienced practitioners of Transcendental Meditation (TM). He found that once they eased into their meditative states, certain individuals could lower their breathing rate, pulse, and blood pressure at will. Benson tried to explain the process from a scientific perspective. After years of study he managed to demystify the TM process and to reduce it to a simple procedure. By repeating the same sound (for example, the word *one* or the sound *Om*) to oneself over and over again in a quiet, comfortable setting, an individual could produce the TM effects. The state of mind this exercise evoked Benson called the *relaxation response.*

Others moved beyond the domain of psychosomatic diseases, to show how mental states could have definite, physical repercussions on other diseases, such as cancer. During the mid-1960s, for example, psychologist Lawrence LeShan stunned many when he declared there was "cancer personality." He suggested that people with certain kinds of personality traits had a higher than average incidence of cancer, an incidence that conventional medicine could not explain.

LeShan was a respected researcher with impressive evidence. Interviews he had conducted with hundreds of cancer patients underscored a behavior pattern. Frequently, they were people who were long-suffering, who preferred to repress their hostile feelings, and who were often typed as having a low sense of self-worth. And, most eerily, prior to their diagnosis, many had experienced a personal loss such as death or divorce.[9]

In the mid-1970s Johns Hopkins University researcher Dr. Caroline Thomas added more weight to LeShan's general thesis as she assembled the results of a study begun more than thirty-five years previously. She and coresearcher Karen Duszinski followed the health of a group of more than thirteen hundred medical students who were Johns Hopkins Medical School graduates between 1948 and 1964.

As medical students, one group had reported they were emotionally distant from one or both parents. More than three decades later this group suffered an unusually high incidence of mental illness, suicides, and death from cancer. Was this all a coincidence? Thomas didn't think so. She continues to monitor the graduates.[10]

This idea that a person's psychological past might affect the physical future received further reinforcement from another long-term study, made at Harvard University and begun in 1937. Called the Grant Study, the project zeroed in on a group of Harvard undergraduates and followed them for several decades after graduation.

In 1967 Harvard psychologist George Vaillant assumed the job of analyzing the results.[11]

In a sensitive and eloquently written book, *Adaptation to Life*, Vaillant detailed some individual cases as well as the general findings made by the study. Although the work emphasized the subjects' psychological development, it also offered other insights, among them that individuals who typically handle the trials and pressures of life in an immature way also tend to become ill four times as often. Immature coping styles are those characteristically used by children and adolescents, including (1) *projection*, unconsciously disavowing one's conflicting thoughts and feelings by imagining them to be expressed in the behavior or statements of others; (2) *fantasy*, redesigning the outer world according to one's wishes; (3) *hypochondriasis*, using real or imaginary disease and suffering to make demands on others; (4) *passive aggressive behaviors*, indirectly aggressive and hostile acts such as procrastinating or deliberately failing; and (5) *acting out*, acting on impulse, from temper tantrums to drug abuse. Vaillant also discovered that men who were considered to be lonely individuals often became chronically ill by the time they reached their fifties.

Although Vaillant did not relate specific personality traits to specific diseases, he demonstrated that immature defenses were not only ineffectual in dealing with life, but unhealthy. By not coping well, people not only were maladjusted emotionally; they were maladjusted physically: they became sick. He also reminded those who read his study of one of the basic truths of medicine. "True, doctors can lance boils and desensitize phobias, remove cinders and anesthetize anxiety," he declared. "But much of psychiatry, like much of medicine, becomes simply supporting natural healing."[12]

"PROVING" COMMON SENSE

On the surface, the long, painstaking work of LeShan, Thomas, and Vaillant reveals little that common sense has not already shown. But common sense is not science. "Knowing" that one's state of mind influences one's body does not prove that it does. The reason that it does not is the problem of explaining how a state of mind can sway the immune system. As one skilled immunologist concludes,

"I know deep down that such influences exist, but I am unable to tell *how* they work, nor can I in any scientific way describe how to harness these influences, predict or control them. . . . In the face of this inadequacy, most immunologists are naturally uneasy and usually plead not to be bothered with such things."

One reason immunologists choose to ignore such questions is because they have enough purely physiological questions to answer. A key to understanding health and disease is knowing how the body's system of self-protection, the immune system, works. Mastery of the subject requires a life's work. Only the central nervous system is more complex. The immune system's complexity is essential for protecting the body from a daily onslaught of microbial enemies. Without it, human beings would die in a matter of minutes.

In the best of all possible worlds, the immune system always manages to use just the precise amount of force necessary to destroy enemies, leaving the unaffected part of the body relatively unscathed. But everyone becomes sick, often because the immune system has either underreacted or overreacted to *antigens,* identifying molecules from microbial interlopers that trigger immune reactions. Thus, diseases are characterized in terms of these reactive extremes:

If the immune system

- is *overactive* in response to an antigen from *outside* the body, ragweed pollen, for example, *allergy* is the medical result.

- is *overactive* in responding to an antigen that is the *body itself*— if the immune system attacks its own body's healthy tissues such as the cartilage in joints—the result is an *autoimmune* disease such as rheumatoid arthritis.

- *underreacts,* ignores, or is unable to destroy an *outside* antigen, a bacterium, for instance, the result could be an *infection.*

- *underreacts* to or simply ignores an abnormal antigen that appears to be a normal part of the *inside* of the body, the result may be *cancer,* in which abnormal body cells are allowed to proliferate unchecked.[13]

These scenarios occur when the system breaks down; fortunately, for most individuals breakdowns are rare. Also, the immune system requires little conscious intervention to perform its function. Like the autonomic nervous system, which regulates vital second-to-second functions, from the heartbeat to the digestive system, the immune system functions without direction.

Unlike the autonomic nervous system, the immune system has been considered an independently operating entity. Therefore, when the studies by LeShan, Thomas, Vaillant, and other researchers were published, they raised a possibility troubling to those immersed in the traditional studies of immunology: They suggested that like so many other systems in the body, the immune system, our main ally in controlling disease, was also susceptible to mental states. That implication flew in the face of everything assumed or written about the system.

It also revived old medical questions and problems. If it is true, as individuals from Hippocrates to David McClelland have suggested, that mental states can influence physical states, medicine has to answer a long list of difficult questions. How does the mind do this? What states of mind have an effect? How do they do what they do? What diseases are susceptible to this influence? If this mental facility is real, can we control it? How? The list goes on.

To deal with these possibilities, any enlightened healer must consider three awesome problems. The first is to have the courage to renounce what is practically medical dogma: that the body's immune system is totally self-contained and outside the influence of any other system in the body. By declaring that the mind can influence the way the body protects itself, one rejects twenty years of findings that indicate that the body's immunity operates without help or interference from any other physiological system.

The second problem is to find exactly where in the seat of emotions and thought, the brain, this influence is wielded. A challenge indeed, since the body's nervous system is the only one more complex than the immune system.

The third problem is to discover the way that the two most complex systems work together. What link or links join these two systems? In short, what is the science behind Fu-zheng?

CLUES TO THE HEALER WITHIN

About fifteen years ago evidence began to suggest that the immune system was responsive to stress. National Aeronautics and Space Administration (NASA) doctors examining astronauts after they returned from space found changes in the white blood cell count that appeared only during the physical and mental stress of reentry to earth. Blood samples taken before the *Apollo* astronauts left for the moon and while the *Skylab* space travelers were in orbit showed normal immune cells. Immediately after their return to earth, both groups had a noticeably lower blood count.

A few years later, another seemingly unrelated discovery supported the NASA discovery. A team of Australian doctors examined the blood of twenty-six people whose spouses had recently died. The doctors were testing the claim that grief is a health risk. Their tests showed that the immune cells from the grief-stricken had lost some of their ability to respond to microscopic immune challenges.

These discoveries would have been little noted if one researcher, psychiatrist George Solomon, had not sensitized the medical world to the importance of such revelations. About the time NASA was studying the blood of its astronauts he was at Stanford University preoccupied with, among other phenomena, the way some people become afflicted with rheumatoid arthritis.

Medically, rheumatoid arthritis is an *autoimmune* disease: the immune system attacks the body's own joints. Again, medically, it is considered a psychosomatic ailment, flaring up or worsening when an individual experiences stress. Solomon was watching the disease closely because he was convinced that a connection between the brain and the immune system existed. This type of arthritis, with its prime emotional factor, provided a good opportunity to test his theory. Since he was particularly interested in the effect of emotional distress on the immune system of arthritics, Solomon tried to decipher the mechanism by which stress affects illness. With the help of a farsighted and courageous immunologist, Dr. Alfred Amkraut, Solomon began to probe for clues linking stress to the immune system.

Together they stressed batches of rats, giving them electric shocks, putting them into crowded cages, before implanting tumors and observing the results. Tumors in a large percentage of the stressed rats flourished and grew faster. Some mechanism was definitely at work. But was the brain a part of the reaction? Logically, it would seem, stress would work through the brain; but this possibility could only be inferred from watching what was happening to the rats.

To test their hypothesis further, Amkraut and Solomon decided to try an experiment they had heard that Soviet scientists were performing. Using small electric probes, Soviet scientists destroyed a tiny area of animals' brains called the *hypothalamus*. They reported that this procedure disrupted the normal functioning of the immune system. When Solomon and Amkraut tried the experiment on their animals, the immune systems of the rats with the burned-out hypothalamus weakened noticeably. Because this result and his stress experiments suggested a link between the mind (psyche) and the immune system, Solomon suggested that this new science be called *psychoimmunology*.

If there were a connection between the brain and the immune system, his work raised more questions than it answered. One particularly obvious and important question was, If the brain can influence the immune system, is there any way to control or direct this influence? Quite by accident, an experimental psychologist from the University of Rochester found out that it is possible.

For years psychologist Robert Ader had been interested in the effects of what are generically called *psychosocial factors*—behavior, attitudes, social environment, personal relationships, the stresses and strains of life—on a person's state of health. Ironically, while he was investigating a seemingly unrelated topic, Ader made his important discovery.

During the mid-1970s Ader had been conducting standard Pavlovian conditioning experiments with rats, teaching them to associate one stimulus with a specific experience, using the same principle that Pavlov had used to condition his dogs to salivate at the sound of a bell. Ader was trying to instill in his animals an aversion to saccharin-flavored water. The procedure was a standard one used hundreds of times by psychologists. After drinking the sweet water, the rats were injected with a drug, cyclophosphamide, which made them feel nauseous. (Ordinarily only one match of saccharin and an injection is necessary to make the rats associate saccharin with the nausea.) During the experiment process, Ader kept having an annoying problem: many of the animals were dying.

At first Ader was totally mystified. The animals were well-fed, healthy, young. Ader reviewed his procedure one detail at a time. It was then that he found the clue: The key was the drug he had been using, cyclophosphamide. The drug was a standard research tool for this kind of work, but he discovered that it had another quality besides causing nausea: cyclophosphamide is a powerful immunosuppressant.

With this new information, Ader began piecing together his thesis about what had happened. By teaching the rats to behave as though cyclophosphamide were in their systems, he not only was conditioning them to hate saccharin; he had inadvertently taught them to suppress their immune systems whenever they drank the saccharin water. Just as Pavlov's dogs salivated at the sound of a bell, even when there was no food in sight, Ader's rats suppressed their immunity even when no immunosuppressants were in the water. For the specially conditioned animals, a taste of sweet water was as effective as a dose of cyclophosphamide. (Ader later discovered that as long ago as the 1920s Soviet researchers had done similar experiments using Pavlovian conditioning. For example, a pair of brilliant scientists, S. Metal'nikov and V. Chorine, conditioned a guinea pig to release antibodies when they scratched its skin.)

To test his hunch, Ader devised a series of ingenious experiments with the help of immunologist Nicholas Cohen, also at the University of Rochester. They repeated the saccharin-cyclophosphamide conditionings over and over again, each time with the same result: the conditioned rats succumbed to infectious diseases more readily. They also became surprisingly resistant to certain autoimmune diseases, a result that also made sense. If the immune system were suppressed, everything it did, including attacking its own body, would be suppressed as well.

In one test of this theory, Ader used a group of rats genetically destined to die of a rat version of the autoimmune disease systemic lupus erythematosus. The rats that received his conditioning training experienced less of the inflammation and lived longer than those who had not been trained. It was an elegantly simple experiment that demonstrated a clear connection between the behavior conditioning and immune changes. Ader published his results in *Science,* the premier science magazine in the United States. When his report appeared, Ader recalls, many people were sceptical. To announce that the supposedly immutable immune system could be influenced at all was heresy enough, but to claim that it could be influenced in a certain direction was more than some could accept. The sceptics tried Ader's experiment and obtained the same results.

Like George Solomon, Ader was convinced that he was moving into a whole new dimension of medical science. And, like Solomon, he was certain that it involved a state of mind (psycho) and the immune system (immunology). But he also believed that any conditioned reaction had to involve the nervous system. Therefore, he took Solomon's term, *psychoimmunology*, and inserted *neuro* into the middle of it, to give credit to the role of the central nervous system in the disease process. The result was the ungainly term *psychoneuroimmunology* (PNI).

During the last ten years researchers from various backgrounds have been gradually drawn to this new discipline. Social psychologists, experimental psychologists, psychiatrists, immunologists, neuroendocrinologists, neuroanatomists, biologists, oncologists, epidemiologists, among other specialists, have all been making contributions to PNI research. For the first time in the history of medicine, there dangles before us the tantalizing possibility of explaining the way the brain and mind make us sick or keep us healthy.

The study of PNI is an endeavor with built-in risks and problems. Partly because of its newness, and partly because it challenges some revered ideas of medicine, PNI has been received with considerable reluctance and suspicion by those with more traditional attitudes. Reactions have varied from indifference to open hostility. For example, Lawrence LeShan found obtaining funding for his research into possible links between cancer and personality almost impossible. None of the standard grant-giving agencies would give him a cent. Eventually he was able to obtain financial help from a small private laboratory.

Some antagonistic feelings continue to this day. In the early 1980s in a section of the National Cancer Institute, the Behavioral Medicine Branch, imaginative PNI work was being performed. Researchers were trying to test an observation made of breast cancer patients: that women with better survival rates were also those who were fighters. They had an aggressive attitude toward conquering the disease and were active in choosing their doctors and treatment. The researchers hoped, first, to confirm whether this theory were true and, second, to find out what could be done to help breast cancer patients deal with their disease more healthfully. By 1982 the branch, only four years old, was disbanded by a new head of that division of the institute. "Psychoneuroimmunological research is not a large part of the Institute and won't be for the present. The issue of how emotions affect cancer is very difficult for us to deal with here" was his cryptic explanation. The head of the project quit and moved on to do research at a medical school with a less hostile attitude.

One casualty of hostility and indifference to the ideas of PNI was George Solomon himself. Although his work had been published in respected science journals—*Nature, Psychosomatic Medicine,* and *Archives of General Psychiatry*—it received little scientific recognition during the 1960s. As a result, after a decade of work in psychoimmunology, he withdrew from the field of research: "I left it for ten years because no one would listen."

Fortunately, the indifference to PNI is fading. Physicians themselves are beginning to see that technology has diluted some of medicine's more humanistic elements, simple parts of the medical ritual, like touch, that have genuine therapeutic benefit. This new consciousness can be found with increasing regularity in the pages of their leading journals, such as the *Journal of the American Medical Association* and *The New England Journal of Medicine.* The message is that our phenomenal progress in medical technology has had a certain cost: "Recently I visited a ten-bed intensive care cardiac unit," mused one physician. "The Faustian soul of modern technology had provided that most touching was mechanical, through electrodes, wires, tubes, scopes, and the like. Medical professionals were rarely in contact with patients. They were [busy] monitoring machines." Another doctor commented: "The specialist-physician is metamorphosing into a technocrat and a businessman. The physician retreats behind the machine and becomes an extension of the machine."

One of the more poignant analyses of the present state of medicine was a brief essay, "Is Medicine Still an Art?" in *The New England Journal of Medicine.* In it, Dr. Truman Schnabel of the University of Pennsylvania School of Medicine compared the way his father, an internist, practiced medicine to typical medical practice today. On the one hand, the medicine of the 1920s and 1930s that his father practiced was primitive and ineffective compared to medical practice today. Patients then stricken with pneumonia and rheumatic fever depended on luck and the strength of their constitution in order to survive.

Yet, Schnabel notes, his father enjoyed a close personal relationship with his patients and managed to perform most of the diagnostic work usually done by specialists today. "To him," recalled Schnabel, "medicine's art lay in a skillful manipulation of the relationship between doctor and patient which, when combined with the logical use of medicine's science, led to the best kind of patient care."

With our current mania for specialists, Schnabel adds, "The sick person seems to have changed. No longer a single entity, the body demanded an expert in each specific organ system." What the technology of medicine gained by this approach, the craft of healing lost. Not surprisingly, says Schnabel, this raises a basic question: Is anyone looking after the whole being?[14]

Of course, good doctors have always treated the total patient. The heavy overlay of tests and techniques may make that task a little more difficult, but a good doctor exerts a real healing power over a patient. There is a real medical power in the healing touch of a caring physician that may mobilize the immune system and ultimately revoke the patient's citizenship in what writer Susan Sontag has called "the kingdom of the ill."[15] It is a time-honored method of healing that predates the oldest drug, the most ancient of therapies. The great frustration of science and medicine is that, until now, there was no way to quantify it, to study it, or even to prove within the rules of science that it existed.

With the emergence of psychoneuroimmunology that frustration is behind us. We are now starting to collect the clues to the identity of the oldest and most reliable unseen ally of medicine. It is the ally who helped David McClelland's healer cure the Harvard University undergraduates' colds, who held Dr. Klopfer's patient from the grave awhile longer, who treated so effectively the disease that plagued Dr. Kirkpatrick's patient. The ally is the healer within each of us. And now, after centuries of being little more than a shadowy presence, a bit of medical folklore, it is beginning to reveal some of its secrets and its powers.

CHAPTER TWO

Best Defense:
The Immune System

ANYONE WHO DELVES into the healing process confronts one of the most complicated systems in the body, the immune system. Immunology, the study of the immune system, is a very young science. Although we have learned more about the immune system in the past twenty years than in the previous history of medical science, we are still far from a complete understanding, because of the complexity of the system and its individual components. Dr. Baruj Benacerraf, Nobel Laureate and professor of Comparative Pathology at Harvard Medical School, has said: "Immunology is one of the more complex, Talmudic areas of biology. The only topic more complicated is understanding how the brain works." Speaking less metaphorically, when asked about his reaction to the challenge of working on the immune system in his research, psychoneuroimmunologist Robert Ader said simply, "I'm scared to death."

Why is it so intimidating? The answer lies in the action the immune system performs: defending the body against infection and disease, maintaining a healthy status quo biochemically. At any given moment several hundred different viruses are lurking within us. If the immunological restraints were dropped, these viruses could debilitate or kill us. Figure 2-1 illustrates the complexity of the process whereby the immune system reacts to antigens invading the human body.

Figure 2-1.

	Results	
	Overactive	Underactive
Outside antigen	Allergy	Infection
Inside antigen	Autoimmunity	Cancer

Generally speaking, the immune system does not let us down. Recently, however, what can happen when this system collapses has been graphically demonstrated by the epidemic of Acquired Immune Deficiency Syndrome, better known as AIDS. This disease went from being a single case in 1981 to a terrifying epidemic by the mid-1980s, when it was infecting an average of five people per day.

The first documented case was that of a young man suffering from Kaposi's sarcoma. What the doctors noted initially was how unusual his case was. Ordinarily the disease, one that begins with reddish-purple blotches on the skin, is rare—only one person in 2.5 million people contracts it. Another unique feature was that this ailment is usually seen in men sixty years old or older. In subsequent victims a pattern began to appear: many were either homosexual males, intravenous drug users, or hemophiliacs. Not everyone got Kaposi's sarcoma. Some developed a form of pneumonia, *Pneumocystis pneumonia.*

By the hundreds, and later by the thousands, AIDS patients appeared at hospitals and clinics, weak, emaciated, their unprotected bodies ravaged by viral and fungal infections. Doctors were horrified to find in AIDS patients everything that could infect a human: bacteria, viruses of all kinds, fungi, and protozoa, so-called "opportunistic" infections. Blood tests indicated what had happened. The immune systems of individuals having AIDS were only partly effective. They could not mount a form of natural self-defense called *cell-mediated immunity.*

The suspected cause of AIDS is a type of virus, HTLV III, which attacks T-cells, important components of the immune system. The immune system has various kinds of T-cells, including helper T-cells that produce substances to boost the aggressiveness of the immune system and suppressor T-cells that can dampen or slow down the activity of other immune cells. A normal immune system usually has two times as many helper as suppressor cells. The immune system of an AIDS victim may have just the opposite ratio.

What this means to the AIDS patient is that his own immune system holds itself back from attacking an invader. Prognosis is poor. Fewer than one out of ten AIDS patients live more than three years after they are diagnosed. Not one is known to have recovered his normal immunological powers.

OUR NATURAL DEFENSE

A normal, healthy immune system, by contrast, is a wonderful phenomenon of nature. Programmed into an immune system is an innate ability to recognize which cells belong to its body and which are foreigners that must be destroyed. It detects foreign cells because of antigens, substances that generate a biochemical response from the immune system. Bacteria, viruses, normal and abnormal cells, and many chemical compounds have antigenic properties.

Another equally remarkable feature of the immune system is its memory. Once exposed to a specific antigen, it never forgets the experience. From one confrontation it learns to produce biochemical

27

weapons specific to a particular antigen. Vaccines, like the polio vaccine, exploit this ability for total recall. That is why, under normal conditions, we can catch some diseases like mumps, measles, chicken pox, and mononucleosis only once in our lives. One exposure, even a small one, to an infectious agent is enough to put the entire immune system on guard against it for the rest of one's life.

Even though this memory is extremely precise, there is one reason why most of us still get colds or the flu year after year: some viruses change their identity slightly over time, a natural phenomenon called *antigenic drift.* That slight change is just enough to let a variant of last year's virus slip past our immunological defenses.

As a general protection against this shifting viral identity, evolution has not only given us immune systems that are adaptable but ones that are sufficiently different immunologically and genetically to offer some natural protection against epidemics. We know that once a virus has modified itself to defeat one immune system, it can race through others that are similar. Viruses spread through strains of mice that are isogenic, or genetically and immunologically identical, more rapidly than through strains that are heterogeneic, or genetically different. That slight genetic differentiation from one animal to another acts as a natural barrier to disease.

We now know that the immune system has two broad strategies for defending the body: cell-mediated immunity and humoral immunity.

Cell-mediated immunity is a defense strategy that uses teams of specialized cells to alert the immune system to the presence of an invader and organize an attack. Cell-mediated reactions specialize in fighting off viruses and attacking tumors; sometimes they interfere with a surgeon's best intentions by rejecting transplanted organs with the same efficiency with which they attack a tumor.

Humoral immunity relies on special molecules, such as antibodies, present in body fluids. Its particular asset is moving quickly against infection—for example, against bacteria introduced through an injury into the body's bloodstream. As the term *humoral immunity* indicates, its rapid response is produced by the body's "humours," or vital fluids, which carry microbe fighters to where they are needed.

The Team: T-cells, B-cells, and Associated Mechanisms

The main players in the immunological arena are two types of white blood cells, or *lymphocytes,* and some related but still not very well understood cells. Together they form a cohesive team with each carrying out a prescribed job. There are immune cells that summon others to attack, there are those that mark the microscopic victims for destruction, and there are specialized immune cells that do the destroying. Still others act more constructively, calling off an attack or cleaning up microbial debris. In all it's a unique system of *yin* and *yang* on a cellular level. Figure 2-2 is a simplified schema of the varieties of immune cells, a skeletal outline indicating the intricacy involved.

T-CELLS

Immune cells are born in the bone marrow and then follow different developmental paths. About half the cells are carried by the blood-stream to the thymus gland, a pinkish-gray body about the size of a walnut located just under the breastbone. The thymus gland is the source of powerful hormones that transform the newborn cells into mature T-cells.

For decades the thymus was the most underestimated gland in the human body. To medical students in the 1960s, for example, the thymus was little more than an anatomical curiosity. Now we know that it secretes hormones and is the site of the transformation of primitive immune cells into fully functional *thymus-derived* (T-) cells.

Carried along in the blood vessels and their tributaries, the *capillaries,* T-cells have the job of patrolling every nook and cranny of the body for foreign, potentially dangerous microbes. They provide protection against cancer, for instance, by destroying abnormal cells before they proliferate. They also help regulate the immune system.

T-cells comprise a major part of the cell-mediated system. There are many different kinds of T-cells. Among the most important are the following:

- *Helper T-cells,* which enhance or elicit the aggressive action of the other immune cells

Figure 2-2.
The Immune System

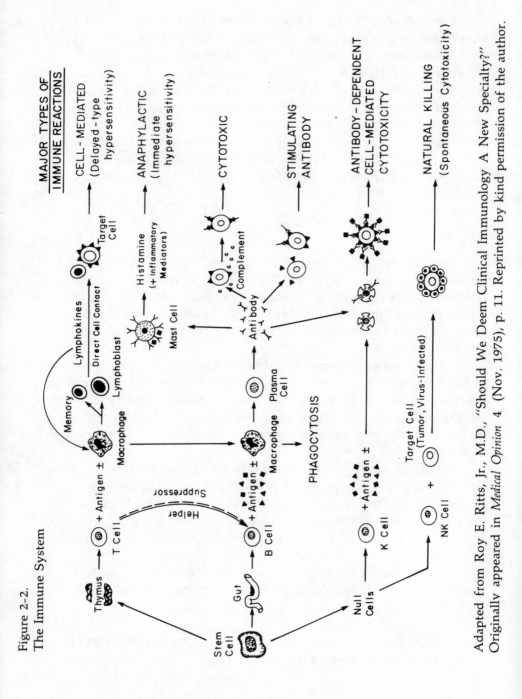

Adapted from Roy E. Ritts, Jr., M.D., "Should We Deem Clinical Immunology A New Specialty?" Originally appeared in *Medical Opinion* 4 (Nov. 1975), p. 11. Reprinted by kind permission of the author.

- *Suppressor T-cells,* which dampen the activity of other immune cells

- *Killer T-cells,* which destroy cancerous and virus-infected cells when properly prepared by a previous encounter with the appropriate antigens.

Helper cells issue the biochemical equivalent of a call to arms, and the suppressors sound the retreat, or, more accurately, the all-clear signal. Both perform these roles by releasing chemical signals called *lymphokines,* which send a message to other immunological cells to attack or, once the microbial enemy has been defeated, to retreat.

B-CELLS

The other type of lymphocyte that plays a major role in microbial self-defense is the B-cell, a prominent agent of the fast-reacting humoral immune system. Of particular importance is the B-cell's capacity to manufacture, on short notice, the germ-fighting substances, *antibodies* (also called *immunoglobulins*). When a B-cell receives the molecular signal, the antigen, of an enemy (for example, a bacterium), it multiplies, manufacturing more of itself, in the process of *clonal proliferation.* The B-cells then begin to churn out antibodies specifically directed against a foreign antigen. At this point the B-cell is transformed into a special kind of B-cell, a plasma cell.

The antibodies are released by the B-cells in the blood and carried by the bloodstream to sites of infection. Antibodies can function in various ways. Some neutralize poisons produced by bacteria. Others coat the bacteria, which attracts scavenger cells, *phagocytes.* These phagocytes then engulf and digest the bacteria.

THE SCAVENGERS

The phagocytes comprise a third important group of immune cells. (Their name, logically enough, is from a Greek root meaning "to eat.") These cells engulf invaders, bacteria, for example, and destroy them. Some are specialized: *macrophages* ("large eaters") are especially efficient at picking up debris. For example, when individuals quit smoking, some residue from the smoke is still scattered throughout the lungs. These cells move through lung tissue, picking up the microscopic debris and carrying it away.

Macrophages signal the immune system of the presence of foreign bodies by bringing such debris to the attention of a T- or B-cell. If a B-cell, already programmed by a previous confrontation, recognizes the substance the macrophage has captured as a foreign antigen, it will begin producing and releasing its antibodies. A T-cell, on the other hand, may call in more macrophages by releasing lymphokines.

AUXILIARY CELLS

Other immune cells warrant a brief mention here. One unusual group are the *null cells,* so-called because they are neither T- nor B-cells. Among the nulls, some of particular interest to PNI researchers are natural killer (NK) cells. Identified in 1974, they are still something of a mystery. One of their particular capacities is that they somehow recognize, without prior experience, that tumors and virally infected cells are abnormal and seek and destroy such cells without harming any normal cells.

A last important group are *mast cells.* Under a microscope mast cells appear as translucent spheroids full of granules. The granules are concentrated lumps of biochemicals: heparin (an anticoagulant), serotonin (a neurotransmitter), and histamine.

Of all the chemicals the mast cell carries, one having particular interest for PNI research is histamine. Histamine causes capillaries to become leaky, letting the fluids passing through them seep out to the surrounding tissue. We also know that suppressor T-cells are sensitive to histamine. They have on their surface microscopic structures, or receptors, that respond to the chemical.

Mast cells are concentrated in the skin; in the mucous membranes of the eyes, nose, mouth; in the intestines; and in the lungs and other parts of the respiratory system. They have also been found grouped near blood vessels in the brain, thymus, and spleen. In its violent reaction to an allergen, ragweed or pollen, the body of an asthmatic releases a torrent of histamine. They play an important part in allergy, an immunologic overreaction. The histamine causes critical breathing muscles, specifically those surrounding the bronchial tubes, to contract; within seconds the asthmatic begins wheezing and gasping for breath.

Histamine is tremendously potent. An extreme lethal example of its potency is anaphylactic shock. Some individuals are violently allergic to the venom in a beesting, with one or two stings setting off a violent allergic response. Once the venom stimulates the immune cells, histamine is released. The breathing tubes, or *bronchioles,* constrict. Gasping follows. There is a sudden drop in blood pressure, and even heart failure can result. The reaction is fast: researchers have seen the deadly reaction occur in animals in as little as thirty seconds.

THE SYSTEM FIGHTS BACK

At any moment of your life your immune system is on the alert. Some cells—phagocytes, T-cells, NK cells—are on patrol, traveling the length and breadth of your body through the bloodstream. Others, such as the B-cells, hover around the lymph nodes and work from a base of operations. In a healthy body, every part of the immune system performs its role with matchless efficiency.

Let us sketch out a little drama. Assume for the moment that while on patrol one of the macrophages encounters a bacterium. If it acts efficiently, the macrophage takes an antigen molecule from that intruder and carries it until it meets a helper T-cell. The helper T-cell recognizes the molecular sign as an enemy.

Instantly, the helper cells send out a chemical signal to the killer T-cells, which begin to surround the bacteria. Similarly, B-cells that were staying close to the nearby lymph glands also pick up a chemical warning of the enemy invasion. Helper T-cells prod the activated B-cells to produce and release into the bloodstream antibodies specific for those bacteria.

Once the antibodies reach the bacteria they attack to form a coating over them. This attracts phagocytes the way blood draws sharks. Before long, killer T-cells and phagocytes are engaged in vicious battle with the invaders. Whoever wins controls the health of the body.

In a normal body the immune cells usually triumph. Once it is clear that the body's immune system has won, another type of T-cell, the suppressor cell, is alerted. It sends out a biochemical signal that in essence calls off the attack. In the aftermath, phagocytes enter and clear up the debris from the battle. The T- and B-cells return to their surveillance duties, with one important difference: there is now a generation of T- and B-cells that remember the intruder.

Called memory cells, these cells are formed in the process of meeting and conquering the enemy; they can recognize this type of intruder should it return. During the next invasion the system will require less effort to attack and destroy the same enemy.

Consider the common skin test for tuberculosis. As part of this Mantoux test (named for the French physician who devised it), a tiny amount of inactive tuberculin, an extract of tuberculosis bacteria, is injected under the skin. If an individual has been exposed to tuberculosis, the immune system, specifically those T-cells that know how to cope with the bacteria, will isolate and attack the tuberculin.

Within two days there will appear on the skin the outline of the microscopic battleground, a small reddened wheal marking the spot where the bacteria have been restricted and defused. This is called the *delayed hypersensitivity reaction:* delayed because the immune system requires a day or so to complete the reaction and go on the attack; hypersensitivity because the reaction causes the site of the injection to become inflamed. If nothing happens after the injection, that nonreaction too is useful, because it indicates that the immune system has not been previously exposed to tuberculosis. (If tuberculin antigen were present, memory T-cells would have reacted against the tuberculin.)

ANATOMY OF IMMUNITY

The preceding is a general description of the process of self-protection. To delve into the immune system in greater depth would be to head into a murky region of bioscience, intimidating to all but a handful of experts. Fortunately, in the field of PNI, immunologists contribute the expertise required for detailed research. The complexity of the research is growing, with new data appearing almost every month.

Another problem is the diffuse nature of the system, which makes it an elusive subject for study. The immune system defies simple anatomical description. The respiratory, circulatory, and nervous systems, as complex as they are, can be described as having a center and divisions. The center of the respiratory system is the lungs; of the circulatory system, the heart; of the nervous system, the brain. Although some regions of the body have important immune functions, the immune system has no identifiable center. It is, as one expert characterizes it with some frustration, "a roving bag of cells without a fixed anatomy."

Various parts of the body play pivotal roles in its self-protection. One is the thymus gland. We now know it acts as a kind of finishing school for T-cells, but for decades it was considered a vestigial remnant of evolution that shrinks with age. During infancy and childhood, it is at its largest. It begins to shrink after the onset of puberty, in a process that continues steadily throughout life. Because of its large size and its location near the windpipe, it was assumed to be a cause of crib death. The hypothesis was that it somehow pressed on the infant's windpipe, interfering with breathing. That misconception, along with the assumption that the thymus was useless, had unfortunate results. Throughout the 1950s doctors commonly recommended that children with noticeably large thymuses receive radiation treatments. The enlarged thymuses were bombarded with radiation. Instead of reducing the risk of crib death by shrinking the gland (as it usually did), it produced a generation of children with a higher than average risk of cancer in the adjacent thyroid gland.

The true purpose of the thymus began to be known during the Korean War, when doctors doing autopsies noted that young men who died after lingering illnesses had smaller thymuses than healthy soldiers killed in battle. Finally, work at Albert Einstein College of Medicine in New York during the early 1960s showed that the thymus was a gland that produced very important hormones: thymosins. Thymosins not only regulate white blood cells, specifically T-cells, but control other hormones and are important in the growth and aging process. The thymus gland, as one immunologist put it, "directs the immunologic orchestra."

To demonstrate the gland's power, one of the discoverers of thymosin, biochemist Allan Goldstein of the George Washington University School of Medicine, used the hormone to treat patients with immune deficiencies. One of his first patients was an emaciated five-year-old girl whose body was able to produce only a meager number of T-cells. As a result she was dangerously susceptible to infections. At the time Goldstein first saw her she weighed barely twenty-six pounds, half the appropriate weight for a girl her size and age. Goldstein gave her thymosin, and within five days her immune system perked up. Her infections began to be cured, and she gained weight. So impressed is he by the thymus gland that Goldstein has called it the master gland of the immune system.

The immune system comprises more than the thymus gland. Just posterior to the stomach is a small, red, oval body, the *spleen,* which contains phagocytes that clear dead red blood cells and other microscopic debris from the blood and acts as a repository for red and white blood cells. Covered with a sheath of muscle tissue, it uses its muscular shell to squeeze out both red and white blood cells as the body needs them.

The Other Circulatory System

In addition to the circulatory system that regulates the flow of blood through the body, you also have within you the lymph system, a separate circulatory system for immune cells. As blood courses through the body, a certain amount of fluid—water and dissolved proteins, for instance—seeps from the capillaries into the spaces of the body tissue. Eventually this fluid, called lymph, is collected by lymphatic capillaries and rerouted through the body's *lymph nodes:* pinkish-gray nodules scattered throughout the body. Concentrated around the armpits and groin, behind the ears, and in the body cavities such as the thorax and abdomen, they vary in dimension from the approximate size of a large seed to that of an almond. As the lymph percolates through these nodes it flows over the many immune cells concentrated there.

In a sense these nodes serve as ambush points for foreign substances, and they release additional immune cells into the bloodstream, which helps fight infection. If you have ever had an infected hand or foot, you may have noticed a tender swelling in your armpit or groin. That swelling signals that a microbial battle has begun and that the lymph nodes are trying to keep the infection from spreading to the rest of the body. Not only are microbial enemies being slaughtered as they pass through the lymph nodes; they are being hunted down by immune cells released into the bloodstream from the nodes.

MYTH OF INDEPENDENT IMMUNITY

For years immunologists have been convinced that the lymphatic system operates independently within the body. "In part because of the complexity of the immune system, many immunologists have concerned themselves exclusively with those interactions within it. The immune system has often been viewed as an entirely independent system within the body," explains neuroimmunologist Linda Kraus of Boston University, "and, with some exceptions, very little attention has been paid to the interactions between it and other bodily systems."

The evidence that the immune system was autonomous, many immunologists believed, spoke for itself. Immune cells placed in a test tube with some of their natural enemies (viruses or bacteria) reacted to the microbes in the glass tube in much the same way as they did within the body. However, recent psychoneuroimmunological evidence and research in other disciplines show that the concept of the immune system as an independently acting biological entity is incorrect.

Work by contemporary immunologists with electron microscopes, radioactive chemical tags, and genetically designed chemical tools such as monoclonal antibodies has established that beyond the realm of the T-cells, the B-cells, the thymus, the spleen, the lymph nodes, and all the other components of the immune system are potent and distinctly nonimmunological forces that shape the development and function of the immune system.

One is time. We now know that the powers of immunity ebb and flow according to internal and external clocks. A normal immune system follows a daily rhythm. One British research team at Nottingham Hospital in England demonstrated this phenomenon in an experiment in which approximately two hundred nurses and medical students received injections of a mild antigen. Researchers then monitored the reaction of each person's body every three hours for the following twenty-four hours.

When they charted the reactions, they found a clear pattern of highs and lows of immunopotency. Typically the immune system was at its weakest around one o'clock in the morning. Thereafter it continued to climb, reaching a high point of strength by 7:00 A.M. In the afternoon and early evening, it reached lesser peaks of potency. This pattern could explain, in part, why drugs that work on the immune system have varied effects at different times of the day.

In one dramatic demonstration of this process Dr. Franz Halberg, a specialist in *chronobiology,* the study of internal body clocks, gave two groups of mice identical doses of radiation at different times of day. After eight days of this radiation treatment, Halberg discovered that the mice that had been irradiated during their active daylight hours were still alive. Those given the nighttime doses were dead. A microscopic assay of the animals' bone marrow, where immune cells are born, showed how profound the effects of timing were. Marrow cells of the mice given the daytime radiation doses were more resistant and had a much lower fatality rate than those of the nighttime mice. Both experiments demonstrated that immunity is not a constant, immutable force. The immune protective mechanism may be on duty twenty-four hours a day, but for reasons that are still not clear, its strength varies over time.[1]

The immune system also changes over longer spans of time. Age is a significant factor in the amount of self-protection individuals have. Newborns and small children do not have fully developed immune systems. Only after about age two does a child have a fully functioning system. Many aspects of the immune system decline with age. After the age of sixty the individual's immune powers, especially T-cell functions, begin to fade. That decline, say some researchers, is one possible reason that the rate of cancer rises with age. The biochemical profile of the system also changes. The bodies of older individuals produce more autoantibodies, substances attacking a person's own body. The high rate of arthritis among older individuals is one example of this process in action.

We are all genetically and immunologically different. Certain immune-related diseases, from breast cancer to rheumatoid arthritis, have strong genetic influences. Other variables that make an immune difference include the following:

- *Diet:* What you eat—substances like zinc, vitamin C—become the raw material for the components of the immune system.

38

• *Side effects of medical therapies:* Cancer patients receiving chemotherapy and transplant patients given drugs that suppress a
patient's immune system.

Beyond all these, PNI researchers believe there are more subtle
influences: a person's moods, feelings, states of mind, behavior,
attitudes, and his coping ability.

Race and sex can make a difference as well. Blacks have
slightly more of one type of the antibody immunoglobulin A than
whites, and women have slightly higher percentages of immunoglobulin M, another antibody, than men. Female hormones have
been implicated in immune changes. Mice that received high doses
of the female hormone estrogen showed a definite decline in their
system's suppressor cells. With some of the restraining effects of
the suppressor cells removed, the animals had overactive immune
systems.

Part of the reason that women have a higher incidence of autoimmune diseases such as arthritis and systemic lupus erythematosus may be that their bodies have an inborn propensity for
more aggressive immune systems. This possibility is still speculative, but the evidence is tantalizing. In one experiment, a group of
mice afflicted with the mouse version of lupus were given high
doses of estrogen. Their diseases worsened. When they were given
male hormones for comparison, nothing happened.

To complicate an already complicated phenomenon, there is no
single, universally accepted technique for measuring the strength of
an individual's immune system. There is no equivalent, for instance,
of the universal technique for measuring blood pressure. For the
moment science has to use an amalgam of methods, each measuring
distinct elements and features of immune functioning and giving a
partial glimpse into the microscopic skirmishes of the body's resistance to invaders. These methods include the following:

• Measurements of cell-mediated immune functions using
blood cells, antigens, and special solutions to simulate in a
test tube the milieu of the human body. Immunologists can
frequently measure the killing or immunosuppressive power
of T-cells, the functions of NK cells, and the proliferative
abilities of T- and B-cells in response to such substances as
foreign cells and antigens.

- Measurements of the levels of immunoglobulins in circulation, a simple test performed with a sample of saliva, blood, or other body fluids.

- Pin-prick tests that measure immune abilities. These include simple procedures, such as immediate-type hypersensitivity tests to detect allergies and the Mantoux test of delayed-type hypersensitivity to an antigen such as tuberculosis.

- Chemical tests that indicate levels of lymphokines.

- Measurements of the percent of various types of immune cells in the blood sample using special markers called *monoclonal antibodies.* These special substances attach to the surface of a particular cell and, since they are known substances, they help identify the kinds of cells to which they attach.

Monoclonal antibodies were devised by two British Medical Council researchers, Cesar Milstein and Georges Kohler, who were awarded the Nobel prize for their discovery. They fused normal B-cells with cancer cells. The result was a prolific breed of hybrid cells able to reproduce indefinitely and produce a specific antibody. With the monoclonal technique scientists can customize molecules that attach to specific receptors in a key-lock style. By releasing the monoclonals into batches of immune cells, researchers can tell from the types of monoclonals that are absorbed what substances immune cells have receptors for.

MAKING THE CONNECTION

A premise of psychoneuroimmunology is that the immune system does not operate in a biological vacuum but in fact is sensitive to outside influences. One source of tremendous interest to PNI is the organ of thought, the brain. If the PNI thesis is true, a line of communication between the mind and the "roving bag of cells" that is the immune system must exist; otherwise, the processes of the mind are irrelevant to those of the body.

We already know from just a few years of research that the brain is a presence in the immune system. The tendrils of its nerve tissue run through almost all important sectors of the immune system: the thymus gland, bone marrow, lymph nodes, and spleen. The hormones and neurotransmitters the brain secretes and controls have an affinity for immune cells. Certain states of mind and feelings can have powerful biochemical aftershocks. The more closely scientists have looked, the more difficult it has become to find an important part of the immune system that has no link to the mind and brain. Now the question is, how does this relationship of the nervous and immune systems work? How important is the *neuro* in psychoneuroimmunology?

CHAPTER THREE

The Brain Connection

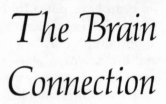

NOT VERY LONG ago, a prominent professor of medicine at a highly esteemed medical school was making small talk with an equally prominent colleague, a psychiatrist. During the conversation the professor of medicine asked the psychiatrist what he was working on. The psychiatrist said that he was studying the relationship between the brain and the immune system. On hearing this, the other scientist looked at him with open amazement. "I can't think of two systems *less* likely to be related," the professor sniffed. He felt he had a right to be disdainful. To suggest that the immune system was regulated by anything other than itself was to utter the medical equivalent of a blasphemy. Even to entertain such an idea was scientifically absurd.

The reasons seemed obvious enough. Ample evidence has indicated that the immune system manages quite well without intercession by the rest of the body. Certainly convincing evidence of its autonomy was the observation that, in the presence of an enemy, immune cells behaved in the same way outside the body—in a test tube, for example—as inside. The message was thought to be clear: the immune system does not work with the brain because it does not need the brain in order to perform its function. It operates on automatic pilot.

Yet here we have Dr. Terry Strom, a widely respected cellular immunologist from Harvard Medical School and expert in kidney transplants, announcing to a gathering of his colleagues: "Despite the capacity of the immune system for self-regulation, a capacity which is beautiful and well documented, I don't think there's any reason to doubt that the brain or hormones may in some ways influence the outcome of an immune reaction." It was a statement calmly made and calmly received by his listeners. But had Strom made such a public declaration ten, or even five, years ago, his colleagues would have responded to it with some shock.[1]

Even today that kind of a sceptical attitude prevails, in part because some scientists have not noticed the avalanche of breakthroughs made by PNI researchers. When a reporter for a leading science magazine interviewed some immunologists about their reactions to the discoveries being made in psychoneuroimmunology, many were not aware the science existed.

Those who have paid attention are observing important challenges to certain medical preconceptions about disease and immunity. The supporting evidence has had a variety of sources: from the surface of individual white blood cells, from painstakingly made expeditions along the elaborate pathways of the body's nervous system, and from the impossibly complicated pharmacology of the body—its opiates, its stimulants, its signal systems—and the mysterious synergy of its elements.

Through incredible patience, ingenuity, luck, and, in some instances, willingness to spend much of a scientific career studying one body chemical, researchers now have some information about the way thoughts and moods set in motion a ballet of hormones, neurotransmitters, and nerve cell activity that has a subtle, but telling effect on health. Today the power of their evidence is such that to deny "the possibility of close links between mental state and immunological reactions ought to be regarded as scientific suicide," suggests European researcher Johan Ahlqvist.

One of the most dramatic demonstrations of the intimate involvement of the brain with the immune system is the series of experiments by University of Rochester psychologist Robert Ader. His accidental discovery was a turning point in current PNI research. By reiterating the Soviets' conclusion that the immune system could be conditioned, Ader sent tremendous shockwaves through the scientific community. Scientists—psychiatrists, immunologists, and others—eagerly replicated the Ader experiment, often in an effort to demonstrate its absurdity. After all, here was a psychologist (albeit with the help of an immunologist) dabbling in a field he could not possibly know anything about.

But they had underestimated Ader. He is a meticulous researcher. In the end, his careful research methods, and the rediscovery of the body of similar research done in the Soviet Union made the difference. Other laboratories had the same results, and other researchers found themselves inexorably drawn to the same heretical conclusions: the model of the immune system as an automatic, autonomous system no longer applied. Years after reaching his conclusions, Ader had the distinct pleasure of rereading the conclusion of his first, controversial 1975 paper with the sense of the prophet who has finally found honor in his own land. "These results suggest," he read, "that there may be an intimate and virtually unexplored relationship between the central nervous system and immunologic processes. . . ."[2]

Thus, PNI explorers have set out to look for what many denied existed: the brain–immune system link, or more probably, links. Certainly there is a temptation to look for a missing link, for what Harvard psychiatrist Malcolm Rogers has described as that elusive "separate mechanism of action"[3] that neatly explains the way the nervous system and the immune system work together. Although the research would be simpler if a discrete mechanism existed, no one believes that there is only one mechanism at work. Medicine, like life, is never simple.

Much of the search centers on the most obvious site, the brain. The notion that the brain might affect the immune system had been around for a while. As long as sixty years ago, experimenters had been flirting with the idea. In one somewhat grisly and nearly forgotten experiment done in 1924, an experimenter took one of his laboratory rabbits, tied off all the blood vessels running to one of its ears, injected an antigen designed to stimulate the immune system into that ear, and cut the ear off three seconds later.

According to conventional theories of immunology, no immune reaction should have resulted. By tying off the blood vessels, the scientist effectively isolated the antigen from the rest of the body; there was no way the immune system could attack it.

Yet when the scientist tested a blood sample from the rabbit, he found in it antibodies specific to those he injected into the animal's ear. Since it was physically impossible for the antigen to travel far enough in the bloodstream to alert the immune system, the researcher reached the only logical conclusion: the immune system could work without the chemical stimulant of antigen circulating in the blood. There is no known way nerve tissue can recognize the approximately 10 million antigens the immune system can respond to. Nerves respond only to neurotransmitters, the chemical messengers of the nervous system. How then did the experiment work? The answer lies buried somewhere in the nervous system.

Much of research has focused on the brain. The hypothalamus has received particular interest because it wields tremendous control over the body chemically, through hormones and neurotransmitters, and through the nervous system. The hypothalamus is a small cluster of brain tissue barely larger than a thumb tip and weighing about a quarter of an ounce. It is situated deep inside the lower midsection of the brain, where it acts as a busy neural interchange.

This small region coordinates a phenomenal portion of the body's activity. The hypothalamus not only transmits but also receives signals over the nervous system and hormonally through the bloodstream. Because of its broad sphere of influence, the hypothalamus could be considered the homeostatic center. It controls specific glands: the adrenal glands and the pituitary. It regulates appetite and monitors the level of blood sugar in the body, as well as the fluid content of blood. It acts as the body's thermostat, regulating temperature control, and is a prime switching center for signals destined for functions controlled by the *autonomic nervous system:* the automatically operating muscles of the heart and lungs and the digestive and circulatory systems.

The hypothalamus is a drug factory. It manufactures and secretes stress-sensitive hormones that unleash a torrent of other body chemicals—epinephrine, norepinephrine, corticosteroids— known to have definite effects on the immune system.

In addition to these characteristics, the hypothalamus has

major immunologic effects. A group of researchers in Central Europe and the Soviet Union were the first to suspect the immune potential of this little patch of brain tissue. In 1958, two Hungarian researchers, Geza Filipp and Andor Szentivanyi, discovered that by removing part of the middle of the hypothalamus, they could protect some guinea pigs from anaphylactic shock. These collaborators found that the animals whose brains had been altered by this selective brain damage showed little reaction to an allergen. In contrast, of those animals whose brains were not altered, ten out of thirteen died when given the allergenic dose.

In the early 1960s word came out of the Soviet Union that one Russian researcher, Elena Korneva of the Institute of Experimental Medicine in Leningrad, had found another quality of the hypothalamus. She could produce different changes in the immune system by selectively damaging different parts of the hypothalamus. For example, when the dorsal, or rear portion, of the hypothalamus was cut, both types of immune response, cellular and humoral, were suppressed.

Psychiatrist George Solomon discovered Korneva's work and repeated some of her experiments, with similar results. In particular, Solomon found that when he damaged the hypothalamus, the thymus gland was also affected: its activity was depressed to a noticeable degree. Since the thymus is responsible for the maturation of the immune system T-cells, the cells that are in charge of immune surveillance and regulate antibody production, this was a particularly interesting side effect. Solomon became one of the first American researchers to suggest that the central nervous system—the brain and spinal cord—played an important role in the immune system.

Where Solomon left off, others have begun. For more than a dozen years, psychiatrist Marvin Stein and his colleagues at the Mt. Sinai School of Medicine in New York City have been studying the effect of the brain, specifically the hypothalamus, on the immune system. In a typical experiment, Stein removed the forward portion of the hypothalamuses of guinea pigs with a small amount of electrical current. He then sensitized the animals to ultrapure egg white, dooming them to overreact violently to the next dose.

When they received the second dose, eight of the ten animals whose brains were untouched died. Of those who had had a portion of their brains destroyed, fewer than 20 percent died. The precise mechanism by which this happens Stein and others are trying to sort out, but it definitely establishes a link between a specific area of the brain, the anterior of the hypothalamus, and the humoral immune response. The message from all this work is clear: damage to the hypothalamus reverberates throughout the immune system. Stein's work suggests that the reverberations take the form of restraining or suppressing the system.[4]

But the hypothalamus is not the only part of the brain implicated in regulation of immune functions. French brain researcher Gerard Renoux of the Medical School of Tours had heard stories that human patients who had severe damage to their neocortex, the brain's gray outer layer, had diminished immune systems. His early work suggests not only that the brain has some influence on immunity, but that different sides of the brain have different kinds of influence.

In brain experiments on mice when Renoux removed a third of the left side of the animal's brain, the body responded more weakly to foreign material. When he removed part of the left hemisphere, the number of T-cells in the spleen, an important collecting point for immune system cells, decreased. (Similar excisions of the right hemisphere had no such effect.) These experiments suggested to Renoux that the left side of the brain has the more direct influence on the immune system.

At this time we haven't been able to isolate specific immune control centers in the human brain. However, we do have some fascinating glimpses of a brain–immune system connection. In studies of people with multiple personalities, Dr. Bennett Braun found that as personalities shifted within his patients, physical changes also occurred. Braun describes the case of a woman admitted to the hospital for treatment of diabetes. The doctors had problems diagnosing and treating her illness because it appeared only occasionally, when a specific personality was in charge. Braun also mentions another case, of a man who had specific allergic reactions to citrus fruit only when certain personalities dominated.

Because these personality changes are more than skin deep—in some patients, personality shifts were accompanied by distinct brain wave shifts—the changes in immune responses implicate the brain as a decisive factor. The question of what mechanism is at work inside the heads of these people remains unanswered. Studies of human subjects linking brain development with the potency of the immune system provide some clues. One particularly ingenious theory was worked out by the late Beth Israel Hospital and Harvard Medical School neurologist Norman Geschwind and a former student of his, Peter Behan, now at the University of Glasgow. Geschwind's hypothesis was that it is not coincidental that people with the reading disorder dyslexia also have a higher than average incidence of autoimmune diseases. The key to the mystery, he said, is the way the brain develops, especially in boys.

Geschwind's hypothesis ingeniously pieces together circumstantial evidence. When Geschwind attended a scientific meeting on dyslexia, someone remarked that dyslexia seemed to run in families. This tendency suggested there was some inherited defect at the heart of the problem. Geschwind remarked that if there were an inherited defect, it might not necessarily appear in the form of dyslexia; it might surface as some other problem.

After the meeting, other participants mentioned to Geschwind that dyslexics' families had a high incidence of other language problems, such as stuttering. They also tended to have a higher than average rate of autoimmune diseases such as ulcerative colitis.

These incidental clues and the phenomenon that dyslexia tends to be more common among boys came together in Geschwind's mind. A crucial piece of information he had discovered in his own research was that dyslexics tended to be left-handed. Geschwind, an expert on brain development, considered the information and wondered what being left-handed, being dyslexic, being male, and having problems with autoimmune disease had in common: "The obvious question is why this association," he said. "You could say that this [autoimmune disease] effect is all psychological due to stress caused by learning disorders. I think this is untenable."

Rather, Geschwind hypothesized that the male hormone, testosterone, and its effect on the brain and the thymus gland was the piece that helped fit the puzzle together. For most people the left side of the brain is the dominant one. It controls the right side of the body and handles verbal tasks—talking, reading, and writing. Because dyslexics are predominantly left-handed and low in verbal skills, Geschwind believed the right half of their brains was dominant. And because so many dyslexics are male, Geschwind theorized testosterone was the clue to their right-brain dominance. (Research on rats and human fetuses showed the right half of the brain tends to be larger among males.) From infancy, testosterone is shaping the growing brain, not speeding up the growth of the right half so much as retarding the growth of the left. The hormone could also have influenced the development of the thymus gland. And, he pointed out, "we know that testosterone can suppress the activity of the thymus gland. Since the thymus is important in the maturing of the immune system, this could help explain the association between left-handedness and immune diseases."

Another possible brain developmental oddity is the basis of an unusual condition called *alexithymia*. First coined by Harvard Medical School and Beth Israel Hospital psychiatrist Peter Sifneos, the term literally means "without words for feelings." There is a group of patients, says Sifneos, who are incapable of giving any detailed description of even the most wrenching emotional experience. Typical was the case of one woman who said of her mother's funeral: "I felt bad but the flowers were pretty."

These individuals are not mentally retarded or nonfunctional people, but for some reason, says Sifneos, they cannot express emotion verbally. Various explanations have been suggested. One, offered by Sifneos and colleague John Nemiah, is that the emotions are felt in the higher levels of the brain, but their expression is prevented by a disrupted connection between the neocortex and the rest of the nervous system. Others have postulated a faulty connection between the two halves of the brain. Usually a bundle of nerve fibers connects the two, but it is possible that this connection and the brain's ability to formulate an emotional statement are defective.

Doctors find working with individuals who have this problem frustrating because they cannot give a more clear or accurate description of their symptoms than vague adjectives. They tend to talk in a flat, robotlike tone of voice and are often quiet, agreeable, even passive in their manner. Sifneos and others suspect that although emotions are not expressed, they are experienced and that it may be that the emotions or reactions to tension and stress are expressed in another way: by illness.

Although she admits that the similarity remains in the realm of theory, psychologist Jeanne Achterberg-Lawlis of the University of Texas Health Science Center points out that the manner of alexithymics is suspiciously similar to some traits of patients suffering from arthritis. "The denial of emotion, the calmness and the repression often described in arthritis patients may stem from quite different origins than those proposed by traditional psychoanalytic interpretations," she has said. Inner feelings and conflicts left unspoken are not unexpressed. They are translated into other signals, such as disease.

Although the neurologic basis of alexithymia has not yet been established, it is now accepted that, regardless of what occurs inside it, the brain has some direct, hard-wire connection to important sectors of the immune system. As part of her doctoral dissertation at the University of California, San Diego, neuroanatomist Karen Bulloch discovered that the thymus of the rat was laced with fibers of the vagus nerve, one of twelve nerves that are wired directly to the brain. The pattern of nerve fibers in the thymus is amazingly consistent among animals, from mice to chickens to humans.

Bulloch's theory is that not only can the brain affect the thymus, but that the thymus needs a certain amount of nerve tissue to function normally and to produce the vital T-cells. As support, she points to the fact that a special strain of mice that have feeble immune systems also have an underdeveloped thymus sparsely laced with nerves. Bulloch believes there is a spontaneous drive from the brain for nerves to make a connection to the thymus. To demonstrate this, in one experiment she enclosed thymus tissue in a porous capsule and implanted it into a mouse born without a thymus. In a matter of time, nerve fibers from the animal's body began infiltrating the capsule, groping for a connection to the missing gland.

Some of her work was confirmed by immunologists experienced in PNI research. In work done at Indiana University, David Felten, John Williams, and others used special fluorescent dyes to trace the pathways of nerves. The networks led not only into areas of the thymus where key hormones are produced, but to the spleen, lymph nodes, and bone marrow as well. Felten also found a network of nerves ending near blood vessels and other areas through which lymphocytes passed, suggesting that they might also influence the flow of blood cells. "Innervation [the growth of nerves] follows the blood vessels into the organs and branches out into the field of lymphocytes," Felten says. "It's a very precise innervation."

Felten's team made another discovery that has genuinely intrigued PNI researchers. Their neurological search showed that many of the nervous system's *synapses,* areas near nerve endings where impulses are sent out, were situated near thymus and spleen concentrations of mast cells, the immune cells packed with lumps or grains of concentrated chemicals. He found whole groups of nerve fibers near these cells, suggesting a direct neuronal connection.

These discoveries highlighted what the group called a *neuro-modulatory mechanism,* which could directly affect the lymphocytes that matured within the thymus and spleen or could affect them indirectly by signaling mast cells to release their potent contents. In short, apparently no major sector of the immune system is without a hard-wire connection to the brain. Understanding the role this mechanism plays in fine-tuning immune reactions will require years of microscope work, but the mere discovery of its existence is bound to be unnerving to traditionalists who doubted that the realms of the immune and nervous systems ever touched.

We have already received some sense of the importance of the presence of the nervous system to the proper function of the immune system. In a simple procedure, a team of Japanese experimenters dosed the sympathetic nervous systems—the systems controlling reflex action in the body—of laboratory animals with chemicals that destroyed the nerve endings. Shortly afterward the immune system went berserk, attacking the body that supported it. Their work suggested that the sympathetic nervous system had a braking action on immune activities. Suddenly the notion that the brain is wired directly into the body's most important means of self-protection does not sound so absurd.

The power of the brain and the nervous system was clearly drawn out around the turn of the century by Harvard physiologist Walter B. Cannon. He was fascinated with the subject of reaction to stress and outlined one scenario of inner events in what he called the *fight-or-flight reaction.* Once the brain perceives that a situation— an IRS audit or a commitment to give a speech—is stressful, that perception becomes a signal from the higher levels of the brain to the *brainstem,* a short bundle of nerves connecting the brain to the spinal column. The brainstem in turn excites the *visceral autonomic nervous system,* the network of nerves that regulate body activities (digestion, heartbeat, operation of glands, contraction or dilation of blood vessels), functions once considered beyond conscious control.

The autonomic nervous system has two subdivisions: the sympathetic and the parasympathetic. The destiny of the *sympathetic system* is to respond to whatever alarm is relayed to it through the brainstem and to help mobilize the body for action. It stimulates blood flow and heart beat and increases glandular secretions. The *parasympathetic system* has a role that is *yin* to the sympathetic's *yang,* slowing the body and helping it to digest its food, and, in general, to take it easy.

When the sympathetic system is activated as part of the fight-or-flight reaction, several events occur almost simultaneously: breathing speeds up to deliver more oxygen to the muscles, the heart beats faster, and blood pressure climbs; the liver releases its stored sugar to help nourish the muscles; digestion slows as blood is rerouted from the stomach and intestines to the heart, central nervous system, and the muscles. The body is literally ready for running away or engaging in combat: fight or flight.

During the stress reaction, part of the sympathetic signal goes to a fatty-looking pair of glands, the *adrenals,* that sit on each kidney. After receiving the signal, the interior of the adrenal glands, called the *medulla,* begins secreting the powerful hormones epinephrine and norepinephrine. Each of these acts as a chemical messenger putting the body into a ready-to-move state.

Most of the knowledge of the brain's effect on the health of the body has come from stress research. We also know that during stress the pea-sized pituitary gland connected to the base of the brain releases the powerful brain drugs, the endorphins. Besides being natural painkillers, endorphins are also suspected of performing other metabolic work: helping us to learn and remember and assisting in regulation of body temperature. They may be the source of the joyful feeling associated with exercise, the "runner's high."

The greatest concentration of endorphins is in the pituitary; at any kind of stress, including everything from depression and bacterial infection to exercise, the pituitary releases endorphins into the bloodstream.

Fascinated by the ability of the brain to produce its own morphinelike chemicals, University of California at Los Angeles (UCLA) psychologist John Liebeskind decided to determine the value of this natural ability to dampen pain. At times, says Liebeskind, feeling pain would interfere with coping with a situation; a wounded soldier who does not feel the searing pain of an injury until after a battle is an illustration of the body's capacity to dampen pain.

Liebeskind hoped to learn more about the system by finding a way to trick the body into producing the painkillers on demand. First, he had to learn a little more about the mechanism that triggered the release of the opiates. In animal experiments, Liebeskind discovered that only certain kinds of stress could summon the natural painkillers. If he gave his animals short bursts of mild electric shock, stress-triggered endorphins appeared. In comparison if he gave them a single, continuous three-minute-long jolt, a natural painkiller was summoned, but it would not be an endorphin. In the vocabulary of brain drugs it was *nonopioid.*

Liebeskind has used this reaction to produce some curious changes in the immune system. When he gave his rats opiate-inducing shocks, certain immune cells, the cancer-fighting natural killer cells, were less active. (This decrease in activity did not result from the longer shock.)

In similar experiments, one of Liebeskind's fellow researchers, psychologist Yehuda Shavit, also found that the tumor-destroying potency of natural killer cells diminished among the rats that had the endorphin-inducing stress.

But these findings were still not definitive proof that the brain opiates caused immune changes. To test the endorphin hypothesis, Shavit injected his rats with a drug that blocks the effects of morphine and morphinelike drugs. His logic was simple: if the endorphins dampened the body's immunity, blocking the body's ability to absorb them, they should also block their immunosuppressing action. That is, in fact, what occurred when he injected the morphine blocker. The animals' immune systems, specifically their natural killer-cells, suddenly became more responsive.

As a further test, Shavit gave the animals a synthetic opiate: morphine. The result was the same endorphin effect. As in the case of the brain chemicals, natural killer-cell potency dropped: the higher the morphine dose, the lower the natural killer-cell activity.

Shavit and Liebeskind decided that the endorphins have an immunosuppressive effect on at least part of the immune system. This effect would explain why, in earlier experiments, they found that the opioid stress made one form of cancer, breast cancer, worse in the rats. Since endorphins are called forth by the brain, the brain also "exercises some measure of control over the inception and development of disease," says Liebeskind.

Still a mystery is the way these opiates do what they do. The brain drugs may work directly on immune cells; they may wield indirect influence by triggering the release of immunosuppressive hormones; or they may have some effect on the nervous system. At this time, any one of the options is possible. One thing is certain— they do not work alone. They are all part of a constantly changing system struggling to maintain an equilibrium, a homeostasis of health.

SMALLTALK: THE BRAIN AND IMMUNE SYSTEM CONVERSE

The idea that the nervous system can influence the immune system makes sense only if it can understand the workings of the immune system. There must be some kind of exchange of information between the systems.

Work with schizophrenics uncovered some common biological denominators. Dr. Allan Goldstein found distinct immunological defects in the blood of schizophrenics. He spotted substances similar to the chemicals found in victims of autoimmune diseases such as rheumatoid arthritis.

Goldstein also found that when he gave schizophrenia victims the tranquillizer chlorpromazine, not only did some of the symptoms of schizophrenia disappear, but some of the microscopic abnormalities in their immune systems did, as well. (Besides its tranquillizing effects, chlorpromazine is also an immunosuppressant.) The same actions that restrain the immune system and diminish the damage done by autoimmune diseases also restrain the effects of schizophrenia on the brain. This correlation indicates that the brain is sensitive to some of the same biochemicals that cause imbalances in the immune system. In a sense they share the same biochemical vocabulary.

If the brain and the immune system have this much in common can they communicate with each other? PNI researchers believe that it stands to reason that they do. For the brain to give intelligent directions to the immune system, it must first know what is occurring. Proof of this hypothesis came from work performed by a

Swiss-based Argentine researcher, Hugo Besedovsky, who showed one way it could be possible by uncovering evidence of immune system–to–brain signals. He first measured the electrical activity of the hypothalamus of a rat's brain. Then Besedovsky injected the animal with virulent antigens. While the rat's immune cells were mobilizing to fight the invaders, Besedovsky carefully watched the brain for any changes in electrical activity.

And he found it. During the immune system's battle there was a definite increase in the firing rate of brain neurons. The frenzied immune activity was mirrored by a more than 100 percent increase of brain electrical activity. Until Besedovsky wired his rat brains, there was evidence that the brain could send out signals to the immune system, but none that it ever received any signals. For the first time, Besedovsky provided that evidence. Some kind of biological conversation between the two systems was not only possible, but demonstrable. "These findings," Besedovsky wrote, "constitute the first evidence for a flow of information from the activated immune system to the hypothalamus, suggesting the brain is involved in the immune response."[5]

He expanded on this discovery when he and other researchers at the Swiss Research Institute looked for changes inside the brain after it received its immune signals. Once immunoreactive material was injected into the rats, the stronger the resulting immune reaction was, the sharper was the drop in the brain level of one neurotransmitter, norepinephrine. This research demonstrated that the immune system could not only get a message through to the brain but could cause some changes to occur. The bond between the immune and the nervous systems was seen to be even more intimate.

Some questions about the way this communication takes place remain. One obvious route is over the pathway of the nervous system mapped out by researchers. Another has been suggested by biochemist Nicholas Hall, who has found another possible brain–immune system chemical connection based in the thymus gland. When the thymus secretes its hormones, they found, it does two things: (1) it hurries along immune cells to maturity as T-cells: the more thymosin secreted, the more T-cells sent out; (2) as already mentioned, it sends a signal to the brain.

The types of messages conveyed Hall does not yet know. Equally mysterious is the reason why the thymus needs to communicate with the brain, although Hall and his fellow researchers have a theory to suggest. We do know that the body has a keen sense of the strength and number of the enemy it is fighting. As part of an exquisitely efficient system of self-protection, thymosin levels rise and reach their peak at about the same time that antibody levels do. Once an adequate number of cells has been called into action, there has to be a method for the thymus to call off the attack. It is Hall's and Goldstein's theory that one way it does this is with a chemical signal to the brain.

THE BRAIN–IMMUNE SYSTEM THESIS

As indicated, the once-revolutionary idea that the brain and the immune system are interlinked is now receiving more and more acceptance. Although not yet scientific gospel, the idea is less shocking than it used to be. Clearly, an idea has attained a certain level of acceptance when a cautious organization like the National Institutes of Health convenes a conference on neuroimmunomodulation to review the current state of knowledge (as occurred in November 1984).

At present, there are two bodies of evidence regarding the linkage of the brain and the immune system. One, largely inferential, includes the following:

- Robert Ader's conclusion that immune functions are susceptible to influence by the brain based on the experiments in which he was able to make changes in the immune system by conditioning behavior.

- Work by the Soviets, George Solomon, Marvin Stein, Gerard Renoux, and others showing that selective damage to parts of the brain's neocortex and hypothalamus can generate selective changes in the immune system.

- More speculative theories of Norman Geschwind, Peter Sifneos, and John Nemiah suggesting that certain structural differences in the brain involving communication affect the course of diseases.

The second body, comprising more direct evidence, includes the following:

- The meticulous nerve-mapping research that uncovered the infiltration of the nervous system into important areas of the immune system: the bone marrow, the thymus, the spleen, the lymph nodes.

- Evidence that the morphine analogs, the endorphins secreted by the brain, have immunosuppressive or immunoenhancing effects.

- Findings showing active lines of communication between the brain and the immune system.

THE LIQUID NERVOUS SYSTEM

The complexity of the mechanism of the brain–immune system connection will become more apparent as we gain information about the two systems. A question yet to be resolved is which system, the immune or the nervous, dominates. Although intuitively one would expect the brain to be in control, the interrelation may not be so simple. Some researchers suggest that the immune system has a level of sophistication that we are just beginning to appreciate. It may operate in the body as a "sixth sense," detecting elements of the environment that elude the other senses. Hugo Besedovsky has gone so far as to suggest that the immune system is an extension of the brain, a "peripheral receptor organ" alerting it to new bodily threats. And psychiatrist Joel Elkes of the University of Louisville has called the immune system a "liquid nervous system."

These ideas are strongly supported by J. Edwin Blalock, a biochemist at the University of Texas. Blalock's microscopic surveys of the immune system have uncovered new surprises, among them that white blood cells can make chemicals that are practically identical to certain peptides that the nervous system produces. Among the body drugs that white blood cells can duplicate is adrenocorticotropic hormone (ACTH), or corticotropin, a pituitary gland secretion that has a major role in the stress reaction.

This capacity suggests, according to Blalock, that the brain is not the only organ directly sensitive to stress; on some level, the immune system has a similar ability to react to stress by using some of the same chemicals as the brain.

As a test of his theory Blalock studied a group of children with pituitary deficiencies who were getting some routine vaccinations. Because of their deficiency, their bodies were unlikely to be able to produce any ACTH when they were stressed. Yet when they received the vaccinations, enough stress to induce a chemical reaction in normal children, their bodies did manufacture ACTH. And the source, suggests Blalock, was their immune system, not their brains.

Given the immune system's ability to sense and react to the world around it, Blalock suggests, "perhaps one of its functions is to serve as a sensory organ." The distinction is that the phenomena it senses are not in the realm of sight, sound, touch, taste, or smell. As Ted Melnechuk of the Institute for the Advancement of Health has put it: "The immune system is a sensory system for molecular touch." The system has an uncanny ability to detect non-self antigen molecules. Lymphocytes can recognize a million different antigens by their molecular shape. Like a language, this recognition ability is dynamic, constantly being updated and revised. When a T- or B-cell encounters an antigen, the antigen prods the lymphocyte to reproduce itself as a clone, or identical group, of cells. These remain in the body for years as memory cells, always prepared to recognize that antigen and to mount an immune response against it should it ever return. If clones fail to encounter the antigen shape for which they were programmed, they gradually die off and disappear. (They were not stimulated to reproduce themselves, and simply diminish in number as each cell lives out its life expectancy.) Despite this gradual decline, the repertoire of recognizable shapes remains more or less constant at roughly a million antigens as new ones are added to the memory banks. In this manner the immune system drifts through time, updating its immunologic memory through a process of molecular natural selection.

The newly discovered relationship between the nervous and the immune systems is bringing medicine back to a more holistic view of the human body. The immune system's unexpected capabilities in working with the brain present new areas for research into the problem of which of the two dominates. The answer may be in the suggestion made by neuroscientist Novera Herbert Spector of the National Institutes of Health. The question is not whether the nervous system controls the immune system or the immune system controls the nervous system. "The answer is obvious," he says, "and future research will make it clear; they control each other."

CHAPTER FOUR

Dr. Ishigami's Message

AFTER TEN YEARS of working with tuberculosis patients, the doctor felt he had learned something important about the disease and the individuals who contract it. In many cases, the disease followed a predictable course, but in others the tuberculosis gradually became worse, contrary to most doctors' expectations, or physically healthy individuals suddenly and mysteriously became ill. The key to understanding such cases, suggested Doctor Ishigami, lay in the emotional life of the patient. "The personal history," the doctor reported, "usually reveals failure in business, lack of harmony in the family, or jealousy of some sort. Nervous individuals are especially prone to attacks of this type, and the prognosis is generally bad." By comparison, in some individuals having more severe cases, recovery followed a favorable course. "These patients are found to be optimistic and not easily worried," the doctor wrote.

"Again, in chronic cases, patients may go on apparently well," Ishigami continued, "until some misfortune happens. This immediately alters the course of the disease. Patients beyond the secondary stage may appear well while nursing their consumptive mother, wife, child, or some such close relative. However, should their dear ones happen to die, with the subsequent despair comes a sudden appearance of severe [tuberculosis] symptoms. . . . These cases may die."

So begins a scientific report on "The Influence of Psychic [psychological] Acts on the Progress of Pulmonary Tuberculosis" written by Dr. Tohru Ishigami of the Ishigami Institute in Osaka, Japan. From the point of view of psychoneuroimmunology, two points of his report have particular interest. One is that a tuberculosis specialist, not a psychologist or psychiatrist, made this report, pointing out a powerful psychological component in what has never been considered to be a psychosomatic disease. Second is the year his report appeared in the *American Review of Tuberculosis:* 1919. Not more than ten years before that, the eminent British physician Sir William Osler noted: "The care of tuberculosis depends more on what the patient has in his head than what he has in his chest."

Osler and this lone Japanese researcher concluded long ago what PNI researchers have been rediscovering: that in the correct sense of the word, every illness can be said to be psychosomatic. Traditionally there has been a select group of ailments, called the "psychosomatic seven," or sometimes the "holy seven": peptic ulcers, hypertension, hyperthyroidism, rheumatoid arthritis, ulcerative colitis, neurodermatitis, and bronchial asthma. The evidence derived from PNI research suggests that this list may be too restrictive. In fact it may be time to retire the term *psychosomatic* altogether.

Both the public and some physicians have used the terms *psychosomatic* (meaning that the mind can influence the health of the body) and *psychogenic* (meaning that the mind can cause diseases in the body) interchangeably. They have lost sight of the true meaning of psychosomatic disease. As Robert Ader suggests, "We're not talking about the causation of disease, but the interaction between psychosocial events, coping and the preexisting biologic conditions."

Several forces shape the origin and direction of illness. Human beings are born with two. The first is our genetic inheritance; everything from eye color to the minute biochemical operations in our brains has felt the impact of our genetic inheritance. Ailments from cancer to heart disease to arthritis can have genetic linkages. The second is our natural constitution. Individuals have inherent weaknesses as well as strengths. Some people just happen to be born stronger than others, part of the luck of the draw.

Individuals have psychological strengths and weaknesses as well. Individual psyches respond distinctively to the psychological equivalent of an antibody: stress. Not everyone responds to the same pressure and not everyone is affected equally by it. Just as some people naturally seem to have sturdy physical constitutions, others seem to be psychologically resilient. Somehow they manage to ride above the major crises of life, while others drown.

At this point let us review what stress is or, more accurately, what we *think* it is. Years after Hans Selye coined the term, no one has produced a universally accepted description. As Dr. Robert Rose, a pioneering stress researcher at the University of Texas, points out, some scientists have referred to *stress* as a stimulus (such as working against a deadline) and the response (headache, ulcer) as *strain*.[1] Others talk in terms of the *stressor* as the stimulus; the response to it is *stress*. A third group defines stress as the interaction of stimulus and response, and others think the word should be dropped from the medical vocabulary altogether. Psychiatrist Dr. Malcolm Rogers of Brigham and Women's Hospital and Harvard Medical School characterizes the problem of dealing with the concept of stress as a "semantic nightmare."

Hans Selye himself considered three definitions before settling on one that he liked: "Biological stress is the nonspecific response of the body to any demand made upon it." Given all the confusion and intellectual haze it is impossible to find anyone working in PNI who relishes using the term, and it is equally impossible to find anyone who can talk about psychoneuroimmunology without paying some deference to it.

And so the term lingers on, for lack of a better one. Whenever it is used here, the term *stress* will refer to the perception of individuals that their life circumstances have exceeded their capacity to cope. In this context, stress occurs within the person, in his or her subjective experience.

There is much less confusion about the internal physiological events of the body during stress. The traditional explanation is that it has a twofold effect. One is the primarily neurological route outlined by Cannon: the signal relay travels through the nervous system. The other is biochemical, involving a cascade reaction of natural body chemicals with druglike effects, each one setting off the release of another.

Hans Selye traced out a path illustrating the extensive involvement of body hormones in stress. In his scenario, when the brain decides it is under stress, it sends a signal to the hypothalamus. That zone in turn secretes a neurohormone called *corticotropin-releasing factor* (CRF), which activates the pituitary gland. Powerful chemicals rush out of the pituitary, among them a large master molecule called *pro-opiocortin*. Along with this, the body produces other secretions, the most important of which in terms of stress is ACTH.

ACTH is a hormone trigger. It, too, travels to the adrenal glands but via the bloodstream, not the nervous system. At the adrenals it stimulates their outer layer, the cortex. The adrenal cortex releases a barrage of hormones, the corticosteroids. Some, such as cortisone, are anti-inflammatory chemicals. They raise the blood sugar present in the body and modulate the body's immunological defenses.

Corticosteroids also act as their own "off" switches. Once released, they make their way through the bloodstream to the pituitary gland. The effect of their reaching the gland is that the pituitary ceases to send out ACTH. Since ACTH is the chemical that initiates corticosteroid secretion, the corticosteroids therefore, in effect, shut themselves down, producing a negative feedback loop. Figure 4-1 illustrates Cannon and Selye's postulated stress pathways. It is a partial representation of the body's biochemical stress routes based on current research findings. In all probability, the total listing of the chemicals involved is much longer, and the interactions are more complex.

For years these interpretations were treated as opposing descriptions of the stress response: Cannon's primarily neurological brain-to-adrenal description (technically known as the *sympathoadrenal-medullary axis*), and Selye's primarily hormonal description (known as the *hypothalamic-pituitary-adrenocortical axis*). Now we know these are variations on a theme. Selye's is an excellent description of the internal events of the body during psychological stress, and Cannon's brainstem–adrenal gland route (the sympathoadrenal-medullary axis) was a better description of the body's reaction under physical stress. The two mechanisms overlap and occur simultaneously. Today we have an even more detailed knowledge

Figure 4-1. The Pathways of Stress

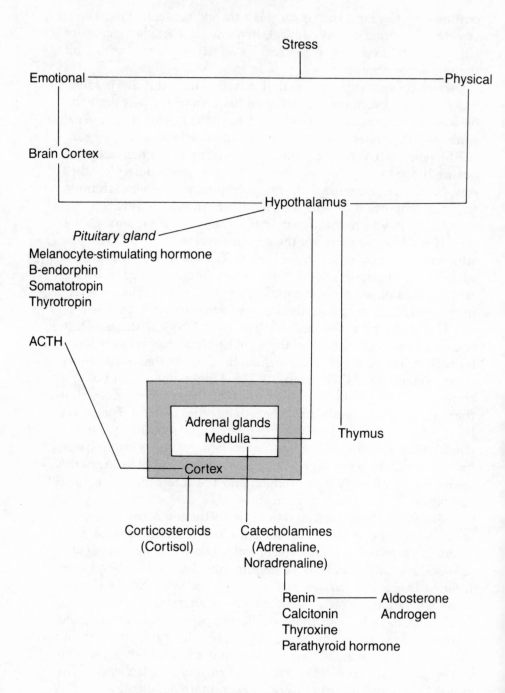

Adapted from "Stress, Behaviour, and Immunity: Animal Models and Mediating Mechanisms" by Myrin Borysenko, Ph.D., and Joan Borysenko. From *General Hospital Psychiatry* 4 (1982), p. 61.

of the biochemistry of stress. Cannon and Selye's modest list can now be extended to include more than thirty neurohormones and neurotransmitters.

Since the immune system is largely a biochemical force, logic suggests it should be sensitive to stress-related biochemicals. The suggestion that high stress situations could affect the immune system has been around for decades. Among the findings Hans Selye made when he dissected his stressed rats was that their thymus glands had withered and shrunk. Since no one understood the importance of the gland at that time, the significance of Selye's discovery was not realized until years later.

Among the first chemicals characteristic of stress studied were the catecholamines: epinephrine and norepinephrine. It has been demonstrated that epinephrine is a secretory response having far-reaching consequences. In fact it is exquisitely sensitive to stress; the extent of that sensitivity was demonstrated by psychiatrist Joel Dimsdale, then at Massachusetts General Hospital and Harvard Medical School, and his colleague Jonathan Moss. They persuaded ten doctors to let themselves be hooked to a small, portable blood pump as they were performing a classic high-stress task, giving a speech, in this instance talking before the hospital's senior physicians during academic rounds.

The pump sipped three samples from each doctor—before the speech, during the first three minutes, and fifteen minutes into the talk. Dimsdale and Moss found a spectacular surge of epinephrine at the three-minute mark, about three times the initial level. By fifteen minutes, it had settled down to about twice the initial level.

Does epinephrine have a specific immune effect? In 1983, a research team from Beth Israel Hospital and Harvard Medical School made a test in which they injected people with epinephrine: "If I just said 'Boo!' to you in a loud voice you would make as much epinephrine as we injected into these volunteers," explained psychologist–cell biologist Joan Borysenko, one of the researchers. This time the results were more complicated. Lymphocytes noticeably increased fifteen minutes after the injections, but after thirty minutes the immune system's potency had started to recede. The overall number of disease-fighting cells had decreased, and with it was a fractional loss of the body's ability to deal with any microbial attack.

Closer examination showed a dramatic increase in a certain

kind of T-cell, the suppressor cell, which holds back the immune system. This increase suggested that epinephrine was capable of unleashing cells whose function is to dampen the aggressiveness of the immune system.

However, during stress a companion hormone, norepinephrine, is also released. To discover its effect on the body a team of researchers from Beth Israel Hospital and Boston University gave a group of healthy volunteers gradually increasing doses of that hormone. The dose was the equivalent of experiencing a mild stress, such as being stuck in a traffic jam. A careful immunological screening showed that after their injection the volunteers had almost twice the natural killer-cell activity in their bodies as before.

Another class of hormones secreted by the adrenals are the corticosteroids. A large body of evidence suggests that the immune system senses their presence in the blood. One emotional state or mood associated with these hormones is depression. Researchers have found that individuals who are depressed also have measurably impaired elements of immunity.

University of Iowa psychiatrist Dr. Ziad Kronfol has performed one fascinating series of studies. For the past few years, Kronfol has been examining clinically depressed patients, those requiring medical attention. Taking blood samples from these patients he used a standard immune test, *mitogen response,* which uses plant products to create an artificial challenge to deceive the immune cells into manufacturing new immune cells. Kronfol has tested blood from scores of depressed patients and has had one recurrent finding: that their immune systems are less responsive than those of normal individuals or patients having other mental diseases. Other researchers have obtained similar results.

We know that the adrenal glands of people who are depressed produce unusually large amounts of corticosteroids, with no apparent biological brake. In depressed individuals abnormalities are present in the functions of the hypothalamus and the pituitary and adrenal glands. Therefore, it is likely that immunity is depressed in depressed people as the result of a malfunction or defect in the neuroendocrine connections regulating corticosteroids. (Chapter Five considers factors—such as bereavement, helplessness, and loneliness—that can bring on such depression.)

Inner states need not be so profound as depression to have an impact on the body. Psychologist Paul Ekman of the University of

California at San Francisco has found that even mimicking emotions influences the body. Ekman, an expert student of facial expressions, has published several studies of the facial expressions of individuals who are in the act of lying. To study the effects of emotional expression in the body, Ekman asked actors to mime the facial expressions for surprise, disgust, sadness, anger, fear, and happiness or simply to relive in their minds a past experience characterized by one of these feelings. By measuring heartbeat and skin temperature, Ekman was not only able to differentiate positive and negative emotions, but to identify the negative emotion an actor was miming through the body measurements. For disgust, an actor's heartbeat and skin temperature dipped. Anger, by comparison, raised both to high levels.

Ekman's discovery underlines the dramatic influence of emotions on the involuntary autonomic nervous system, which directs so many vital physical and hormonal processes. And since the involvement of the nervous system in the regulation and functioning of the immune system is becoming increasingly apparent, this point has particular interest to the PNI researcher. In themselves emotions are not necessarily significant physically. A flash of anger and a moment of despair are fleeting events psychologically and physically. When these emotions linger and become long-term states of mind, they are not so inconsequential, especially when they are negative feelings. The longer a negative feeling persists, the more troublesome it may become.

THE CONTROL FACTOR

It has become popular folklore and, with more careful investigation, a medically documented fact, that bereaved people, widowers in particular, become ill more readily than other individuals. University of Colorado psychologist Steven Maier speculated that because bereaved persons had no control over their loss, they felt helpless and were highly stressed. To duplicate this sensation of helplessness with laboratory animals, Maier and his colleague Mark Laudenslager connected two groups of rats to a simple device that gave mild shocks to their tails. Rats were tested in pairs, each receiving the same shock at the same time. Their situation was identical in every respect but one: one of the rats could switch off the shock to his own and his partner's tail by turning a small wheel. The other rat's helpless destiny was to wait until his colleague learned to operate the control to turn off the electricity.

Among the helpless group Maier found that white blood cells were noticeably more listless than those of the rats with the power of control over the switch. Since the amount of shock received by each animal was identical, there could be only one explanation for the drastic immune differences: loss of control.

Psychiatrist Dr. Martin Reite discovered a similar phenomenon in monkeys. As part of his research at the University of Colorado he has been observing the deep-seated effects of the awful trauma of separating an infant from its mother. Reite put six-month-old monkeys into a cage separate from their mothers. The animals exhibited all the outward expressions of depression and malaise in the mother's absence. Going beyond the skin-deep impressions, Reite took blood samples before and after separation and ran an immune test that checks the white blood cells' ability to proliferate. After separation there was a definite reduction in blood cell activity.

Experiments by psychologist Martin Seligman at the University of Pennsylvania set the scientific stage for much of this work. For the past twenty years Seligman has been making a study of the effects of helplessness on animals and people. His thesis is, very simply, that helplessness is a learned reaction. He is convinced that at one point or another in life some people encounter a stressor or an experience that is more than they feel they can handle. After repeated attempts to cope, they sink into a deep state of despair and eventually simply give up. Individuals no longer attempt to cope with the challenges and problems of the environment because, Seligman suggests, they have learned that nothing they do makes any difference.

The idea came to Seligman when he had been working with dogs in an experiment requiring that they be suspended in a *Pavlovian hammock*, basically a cloth strap that allowed dogs to be restrained as gently as possible. While dangling, they were trained to associate the sound of a certain tone with an electric shock. After a few sessions in the hammock, it became evident to the animals that when the tone sounded, a painful shock would soon follow.

After the hammock conditioning, the next step was to put these same animals into a *shuttle box*, a small chamber in which half of the floor is electrified. When Seligman put an unconditioned dog into the shuttle box and shocked it, usually the animal ran around frantically until it accidentally jumped over a low barrier to the shock-free side. After a while the dog was skilled at avoiding shock. It sat close to the divider and at the first tingle of electricity nonchalantly hopped over the barrier to safety.

When Seligman put one of his hammock-conditioned dogs into the shuttle box, however, the result was "bizarre."

This dog's first reactions to shock in the shuttle box were much the same as those of a naïve [unconditioned] dog: it ran around frantically for about thirty seconds. But then it stopped moving; to our surprise, it lay down and whined. After one minute of this we turned the shock off; the dog had failed to cross the barrier and had not escaped from the shock. On the next trial, the dog did it again: at first it struggled a bit, and then, after a few seconds, it seemed to give up and to accept the shock passively. On all succeeding trials, the dog failed to escape.

It is Seligman's thesis that the whimpering, shocked dog is a metaphor for those who succumb to stress they consider overwhelming. This sense of helplessness has its emotional fallout. Those chronically afflicted with it typically become passive. They have no appetite for sex or food and are depressed and in a constant state of worry and fear.

Physically, helplessness can be equally devastating. Ulcers and other stress-related diseases can occur in the wake of it. The combination of a weakened physical condition and overwhelming emotional stress can sometimes be lethal. Seligman mentioned one instance in which a man, an asthmatic, had been talking on the phone with his mother when she disowned him in a most melodramatic way. He had been trying to start his own business, and his mother, jealous at being excluded, essentially cursed it. She told him that without her help he would never succeed in his new venture. Within an hour of the phone call in which she delivered this dire prediction the man succumbed to a lethal asthma attack.

Recently Seligman has begun to apply his theory more specifically. He and two other University of Pennsylvania researchers, Madeline Visintainer and Joseph Volpicelli, have found that cancer cells injected into rats that had helplessness-inducing shock produced tumors twice as often as in rats that could control the identical shocks.

Psychologist Jay Weiss of Duke University has followed Seligman's and Maier's work closely and has duplicated some of their experiments, obtaining the same results. Weiss has proposed a biochemical description of the physiological events occurring inside these animals. He took a group of rats and made them helpless by pushing them nose-first into a wire mesh funnel so that they were totally restricted. While in this position, they received small shocks of electricity, shocks they could not control, on their tails. Weiss's rats showed the same lassitude, the same animal equivalent of despair, that Seligman's dogs demonstrated.

Weiss thinks that a "motor activation deficit" occurred. The helpless rats simply could not get their muscles to function normally after a session of helplessly experiencing shocks. Weiss concludes that the reason for the reaction is based on his discovery that the brains of these rats were seriously depleted of norepinephrine, a prime neurotransmitter needed to keep the body's nervous system operating smoothly. In trying to respond to a stress, the body generates increasing quantities of this natural brain drug in its standard fight-or-flight reaction. But any body, whether a rat's, a dog's, or an advertising executive's, can release only so much. After a while, it needs a rest to produce some more.

Therefore, Weiss suggests that one reason animals and people are unable to respond beyond a certain point under stress is that their reservoirs of norepinephrine, and possibly of other biochemicals vital to normal body activities, are drained dry in response to the excessive challenge. And since the body requires neurotransmitters such as norepinephrine to enable its muscles to function properly, being drained of these important chemicals prevents the body from reacting strongly to a stressful situation. Thus, the rat has not necessarily lost the will to respond, but the physical capacity to respond. Describing an individual as feeling drained by a stressful experience may be more accurate than metaphorical.

The studies just described are some of the strongest evidence for the way reaction to stress affects—in these instances, suppresses—the body's immune system. Dr. Ziad Kronfol suggests that since bereavement and depression have similar symptoms, it is possible that the biochemical processes of a depressed person may also occur inside a widow or widower. Kronfol postulates that depression, specifically the corticosteroid havoc wreaked by depression, has a devastating immunological effect on some individuals.

Since one of the premises of much of the early stress research was that many events in a person's life, minor as well as major, influence health, it is interesting to speculate whether the lesser crises of life also affect the human immune system. Volunteers from the halls of academia, traditionally fertile ground for stress research, participated in research into a possible association. Students have often been subjects of stress research, first, because they are members of the academic environment, and, with their constant schedule of exams and papers, they can be expected to be experiencing pressure at any given time.

With the help of a team of researchers, Locke examined a group of Harvard undergraduates to determine the effect of stress on their immune status. As a yardstick for gauging stress levels, he used a customized version of the forty-three-item Holmes-Rahe scale, adapted to include the life crises students would more likely face (including number-rated items such as failing a course and changing majors). As a parameter of immune system strength the activity of cancer- and virus–fighting natural killer cells was measured.

In addition, he quizzed the students about their inner emotional experiences: whether they were depressed, the amount of anxiety they were feeling, and the intensity of those feelings. Those who reported that their negative feelings were not very intense were tagged as "good copers," and those who said they were tremendously depressed by or anxious about their problems were characterized as "poor copers." By matching the natural killer-cell level of each person's immune system against the subjective report of feelings, he hoped to correlate individuals' ability to cope with life stress with their immune system function.

He found distinct differences between the vitality of natural killer cells in the good copers and those of the poor copers. Poor copers typically had more depressed natural killer-cell activity; by comparison, good copers, who claimed to feel little distress, had more active natural killer cells.

Psychologist Janice Kiecolt-Glaser and her colleagues at the Ohio State University College of Medicine had similar results in studies of another high-pressure academic group, medical students.[2] As part of her tests Kiecolt-Glaser took two blood samples, one a month before final exams and a second on the first day of exam

week. To find out what was going on in the students' minds as well
as their bodies, she administered mood survey tests in which subjects were to describe their predominant attitude and moods, for
instance, characterizing how lonely they felt. The study produced
evidence that even relatively minor life stresses leave their mark on
the immune system.

Two major findings resulted from Kiecolt-Glaser's work. First,
even the tension and anxiety of a stress as routine as taking an
examination had a distinct immune effect. Further, the exam takers
who said they felt high stress had fewer active natural killer cells.
The second finding that interested Kiecolt-Glaser was that subjects
who said they felt extremely lonely were also the students whose
immune systems registered the greatest impairment. Since this loneliness factor seemed to be a distinct component affecting the immune system, Kiecolt-Glaser now wonders whether loneliness
might also be an important factor in the way bereavement affects
the health of some widows and widowers.

In studying a variation on the experience of bereavement, Isra-
eli scientists from the Weizmann Institute of Science and Jerusa-
lem's Kaplan Hospital found that among women who had lost
unborn children through either spontaneous or medically induced
abortions, their attitude rather than the kind of abortion that occurred made a critical immune difference. Psychiatric tests divided
the women into two groups: the nonaccepting ones, who found it
hard to accept the consequences of their abortion, regardless of the
way it happened, and the ones who were less anxious, less upset.
The reactions of the nonaccepting group, noted the scientists, were
very much like those of a person grieving the death of someone
close.

Of special interest was the immune system profile of each
group. Those women who were having more difficulty coping with
the loss of their child had more feeble T-cell strength than those
who had coped with the loss adequately. Those of the nonaccepting
group who were most depressed also registered the greatest jolt to
their systems. Like the others mentioned—the poor copers and Kiecolt-Glaser's lonely students—those individuals had a definite shift
in the immune system. According to the scientific evidence change
in the immune system corresponded not to the two kinds of abortions, but to the inner reactions of the women to the abortions. That
inner experience had a definite influence on the body.

More than sixty years has elapsed since Dr. Ishigami reported his classic observations of his tuberculosis patients, but only now does it appear that we are beginning to understand the reasons and ways that a mood or attitude manifests itself within the body's system of defense. So far, there is some evidence of the way the biochemical aftershock of emotional states sways the immune system. But the important point is that life's major, traumatic events are not the only ones that can do this. Response to minor daily insults and hassles is also involved in the process.

The encouraging aspect of this realization is that individuals are not helpless targets for every stressor that comes their way. Research suggests that the way individuals perceive these onslaughts on their sanity and health makes a great difference to the body's response. Like the rest of the body, the mind has its own homeostasis and struggles constantly to maintain an emotional balance, to keep peace and health within.

Both animals and people demonstrate a wondrous and heartening flexibility in adapting to stressful situations. One experiment that illustrated this flexibility was made by the learned-helplessness expert, psychologist Martin Seligman. Seligman and his colleagues transplanted tumors into groups of rats before they received shocks that they either could or could not control. In addition, some received brief shocks, to simulate *acute,* or short-term, stress; others received longer jolts simulating *chronic,* or longer-lasting stress.

The rats that received uncontrollable but brief shocks developed tumors twice as often as rats with control. Rats that received uncontrollable and long shocks had about the same pattern of reaction. When Seligman tried a variation on the experiment he obtained a distinctly different reaction.

He took another group of rats that had already been given long-term shocks, both controlled and uncontrolled, and implanted tumors into them after they had been through their shock course. No noticeable difference in the way the tumors grew in the long-term shock group appeared. Whether or not they had control seemed to be irrelevant. But when he implanted tumors into the rats given the brief shocks of both types, their tumors grew more rapidly.

What do these results indicate? Seligman suggests that short-term, acute stress may weaken an immune system, whereas long-term stresses cease to have a negative effect beyond a certain point.

Not only may individuals become accustomed to a relentless shock; they may even become stronger because of it. Like so many other ideas in this field, the idea awaits proof, but this and other studies underscore the way the interplay of various influences directs the effect of stress. As Harvard psychologist-biologist Joan Borysenko suggests, "The nature of stress, its duration, and the interval between the stress and the immune measurements are extremely important."

The inner experience of stress shapes the direction and the force with which it jolts the system. Although two people in the same place at the same time may ostensibly have the same experience, the significant influence on its outcome is the person's perception of the event: the individual's subjective degree of control, capacity to manage the situation, and in Ishigami's phrase, personal history. The way that inner experience, according to some of the research previously discussed, modulates a stressor makes a profound difference on its outcome, all the way to the cellular level. Bombarding this individualized stress reaction are stressors with greater and lesser ferocity. Researchers in psychoneuroimmunology are investigating what they are and what they do.

CHAPTER FIVE

The Real World Factor

DURING THE 1960s, while most of his colleagues were doing research on the biochemical effects of stress on lab rats in the cloistered settings of a university, psychiatrist Peter Bourne was studying the ultimate research animal, the human being, facing the ultimate stress: almost-certain death or mutilation.

Bourne was a psychiatrist in Vietnam. In the late 1960s he was visiting an isolated military outpost near the Cambodian border that was staffed by a twelve-man Special Forces "A" team, an elite group of U.S. Army Green Berets. Bourne had permission to do biochemical stress research on men in battle. An important part of his equipment was a small, gas-powered field refrigerator to store the material for study, urine samples from each member of the team. He planned to analyze them for 17-hydroxycorticosteroid (17-OHCS), a chemical secreted by the adrenal glands during times of stress.

From a researcher's perspective, the group was ideal. The men had a great deal in common. All were professional soldiers with combat experience. Each was highly trained for a specialized job— demolitions expert, medic, radio operator—and worked cohesively with the others as part of a team.

While Bourne was at the camp, the team intercepted an enemy radio message on May 10 that indicated that some time between May 18 and May 22, probably May 19, a contingent of Viet Cong planned to overrun the outpost in a massive ground attack. Highly trained and all combat veterans, the men knew exactly what to do, and each moved into action to prepare for bloody battle. The enlisted men laid out additional land mines, reinforced the camp's barbed-wire defenses, checked ammunition supplies, and prepared a medical bunker for the casualties. The officers were on the radio with command headquarters constantly, keeping their superiors informed of new developments and coordinating their defense plans with other military units in the area. Bourne, meanwhile, continued to collect his samples. The frenzy of preparation became even more intense as the attack day drew nearer. The group expected nothing less than a reprise of an Alamo-caliber battle. As Bourne checked his samples, he found that stress levels, as measured by 17-OHCS, were divided neatly between the enlisted men and the officers. As the date of the projected battle approached, the level of the stress chemical climbed in the officers, reaching a high on May 19. Besides the danger of battle, the officers faced another kind of pressure: their management of this attack, assuming they survived, would affect future assignments and promotions for the rest of their military careers. The 17-OHCS levels of the enlisted men, by contrast, dropped, reaching a low on attack day. On May 19 no attack occurred. Neither was there an attack on May 20, nor on any of the other expected days. It was a false alarm.

In the meantime Bourne had to explain the clear differences of reactions between the enlisted men and the officers. He reached the following conclusion. For the enlisted men, preparing for battle was a matter of following orders and performing well-rehearsed tasks: checking perimeter defenses (mines and barbed wire), getting the weapons ready and into position, setting up a first-aid station for the inevitable casualties. This role gave them a clear-cut way to manage the stress of facing battle. In fact, as camp activity increased, Bourne noticed, the level of the stress chemical decreased.

The officers, on the other hand, not only had no physical outlets for their stress and anxiety but also their situation was more complex. As attack day approached, their duties became more psychologically demanding. They had to worry constantly about their men, about holding the camp, and about putting in a good military performance. They had to make command decisions hourly and at the same time fend off the sometimes useless suggestions of superiors dispensing their advice blindly from a command post forty miles away.

To a man, every officer's stress-hormone profile showed an increase in stress during the preattack period. As mentioned, all the enlisted men's dipped, with one exception: the radio man, whose level of stress chemical mimicked the officers'. The reason, suggests Bourne, was that he not only had no physical outlet for his stress but because his job required being at the side of the camp commander. He was the one enlisted man most directly involved in the tensions and pressures of command decisions.

Bourne's wartime experiment provides an apt metaphor for what used to be thought a simple matter: measuring the psychological shocks of an event. Here was a single event, happening to a group of people similarly trained and experienced, all in the same place, all in the same danger. Because a few of them had to deal with another dimension of problems, commands from headquarters, they were catapulted into another level of stress. And this situation, in a certain sense, is what the PNI expert has to sort out: the way circumstances, inside and outside a person, interact to affect response to a given situation and, ultimately, to disease. At this point researchers think that they know what happens inside the brain and body during stress: the specific biochemical and neurological switches. However, they need to form a clearer picture of the stimuli that trip those switches. Once they do, it will be possible to start moving, as some already have, in the direction of learning to use PNI insights for self-protection.

THE NEW MYTHOLOGY OF STRESS

Part of the effect of the new awareness produced by PNI research has been the demythologization of traditional understandings about stress. In fact, most PNI experts have tried to avoid that term altogether and instead talk about *psychosocial factors* in disease. These factors cover a broad range—from an individual's life-style, job, and place of residence, to that individual's sex, race, social status, cultural background, and personality.

Science and medicine are starting to realize some conclusions in the wake of PNI research. One, already mentioned, is that the traditional concept of psychosomatic disease is outdated, and the term *psychosomatic medicine* is redundant. To continue using it perpetuates the Cartesian myth of a mind-body dualism in medicine. More than thirty years ago, Alexander, one of the guiding lights in psychosomatic medicine, concluded: "Theoretically every disease is psychosomatic, since emotional factors influence all body processes through nervous and humoral pathways." We now know that stress is an important element in approximately forty diseases and a contributing factor in at least a dozen others.

STRESS AND THE IMMUNE SYSTEM: TALK TO THE ANIMALS

The evidence that stress has significant impact on more than the so-called psychosomatic seven is based on direct observation of animals and humans under duress. Since deliberately subjecting humans to potentially unhealthy duress is unethical, PNI experts have used their experimental ingenuity to design high-stress ordeals to test the vulnerability of animal immune systems.

The history of research in this field involves myriad studies in which rats, mice, monkeys, and guinea pigs were restrained, crowded in cages, and exposed to their natural predators in the interest of studying the effects of these stresses on their bodies. In what is now considered to be a minor masterpiece of ingenious PNI experiments, cancer researcher Vernon Riley of the Pacific Northwest Research Foundation meticulously demonstrated that even a relatively benign stress could weaken an animal's disease resistance.

In one series of tests Riley used a strain of mice genetically programmed to develop breast tumors. Half lived in a standard laboratory holding room and half lived in carefully designed low-stress quarters: a soundproof environment where each mouse had comfortable individual quarters. Life was made as easy and as peaceful as Riley and his staff could make it for the mice.[1]

He had more than the comfort of the animals in mind. He knew that those who studied the immune system noted that even minor stresses could skew their findings. It became part of the ritual of research that lab animals had some time after shipping to adjust to their new surroundings before they were used in experiments. For example, Ronald Herberman, an immunologist at the National Cancer Institute, routinely allows mice shipped to him to rest for two weeks before he uses them. Given the fine cellular scale on which he works, the stress of shipment would inevitably affect the accuracy of his immunological tests.

For these reasons, Riley wanted to eliminate as many unplanned stresses as possible. Rats and mice are typically kept in crowded cages in noisy rooms where lights are left on or turned off and on at all hours and chaos reigns. Technicians wander in and out, and animals are frequently jostled, moved around, or removed to be tested or killed for examination on the dissecting table. Riley decided that he needed a group of animals who had been coddled in exceptionally benign surroundings and whose systems had been untouched by the disturbances and confusion of the standard holding room. The animals had separate cages, lived in a temperature-controlled environment, and were cared for by specially trained staff members. Riley even took the precaution of making sure they were isolated so none could even pick up the scent of pheremones, subtle chemical signals given off by animals (and humans) under fear and stress.

Once he had an established colony of quietly raised animals, Riley subjected the mice to a series of stress experiments. All were mice bred to contract a certain kind of breast cancer. Riley wanted to determine whether applying limited outside stress could affect the growth of the cancer.

Rotational stress in Riley's study involved placing the mice in a cage attached to the top of a multispeed record turntable and spinning them around. He divided his mice into four groups. One group was put into cages and on the turntable at 16 revolutions per minute (rpm). The second group was spun at 33 rpm, and a third at 45 rpm. The fourth group was spun at 78 rpm. The fifth group was left to live the good life in the luxurious cages.

The mice were remarkably adaptable. Some managed quite well, eating, drinking, even mating at 16, 33, 45, and 78 rpm. The insides of their bodies told a different tale. Riley found that the higher the revolutions per minute, the larger the tumors an animal was likely to have. The elegant features of the experiment were that not only did the stress of life on the turntable have a definite effect on the way the animals' bodies handled the congenital tumors, but it showed a neat correlation between the degree of stress and the speed with which the disease developed.

Doing similar work, another experimenter, Andrew Monjan, then at Johns Hopkins University's Department of Epidemiology, and his colleague M. I. Collector obtained more complex results. This time, instead of using a turntable, the two researchers blasted the mice with five seconds of a 100-decibel noise once a minute for three hours a night. (This procedure was not so inhumane as it might sound: the 100-decibel level is approximately equivalent to the exposure a rock fan sitting in expensive seats about ten feet from the stage receives.)

Monjan and Collector also found signs that the strength of the mouse's immune system (measured by the rate at which white blood cells divided when exposed to special chemicals) diminished at first. But after two weeks, the animals' systems made an about-face. They not only regained their old potency but actually seemed to grow stronger under the stress of the loud-noise tests.

Like Riley's work, Monjan's demonstrated that stress has an impact on the immune system, with stress effects changing over time. It suggests a two-part, or *biphasic,* response to stresses, registered in the ebb and flow of certain chemicals and immune substances. Monjan's research further implies that, if prolonged, stress saps the vitality of an individual's immune system. Yet the pattern showed that after days, even weeks, of enduring a stress, the body may still rebound. However, we speculate that if the stress is unrelenting, continuing for months or years, eventually the immune system loses this resilience. It may suffer serious damage, and the animal, or human, may slip into a vulnerable state of immunocompetence.

Unfortunately the effects of stress are not so straightforward. Other experimenters have shown we cannot necessarily draw the simple equation long-term stress = long-term immune damage. As just one example, Harvard Medical School psychiatrist Malcolm Rogers and his colleagues at Brigham and Women's Hospital subjected some arthritic mice to a mouse nightmare: placing a cat beside the animals' cages and letting it stare in while the mice scrambled around in terror. This was repeated day after day. Paradoxically as a result of this, the terrified mice seemed to have an increased resistance to arthritis.

THE HUMAN FACTOR

To identify and analyze the mechanisms the preceding results indicate, scientists extend their focus to the ultimate research animal, humans. The usefulness of data derived from animal research and their relevance to humans is limited. Furthermore, subjecting humans to the types of procedures applied to animals is unethical. Generally PNI research has used the kind of approach Peter Bourne used, namely studying people already under some kind of naturally occurring stress.

One of the great frustrations of real-life studies is the problem of excluding unknown variables, the research equivalent of pollution, from the tests. Because there is no certain way of knowing every variable at work in a person's life, researchers must devise environments as totally controlled as is scientifically possible and ask subjects to live in them for a while. One Swedish research team used that technique in one of the few attempts to construct a carefully orchestrated high-stress world.

Experimenters at Sweden's Karolinska Institute, an internationally known stress research laboratory, studied human volunteers who spent days in laboratory worlds where practically every moment is calculated to be stressful. In a famous series of tests made over a three-day period, experimenter Jan Palmblad asked a group of people to shoot at a small moving tank using a rifle that fired a beam of light. The tank had a light sensor that registered a hit from the beam. For every direct hit subjects were rewarded with 90 decibels of realistic battle noise. Individuals were required to shoot at the tank around the clock, for two hours at a time. And they had to do it with no sleep, with the stress of the battle noise and with restricted access to the basic necessities (meals and bathroom visits were rigidly scheduled). This schedule was the focal point of the subjects' lives. Always present were the pressure to perform well, plus the stresses of loud noise, and sleeplessness.

Palmblad was especially curious to determine whether the ordeal had any effect on people's immune systems. At the end of the test he had his answer. The immune cells of the sharpshooters lost some of their ability to kill bacteria. He also found high levels of stress hormones, such as epinephrine. In theory, there was a clear relationship between his laboratory ordeal and the microscopic changes in the immune system.[2]

To demonstrate this relationship, Palmblad might have carried the experiment to its logical (and unethical) conclusion by exposing the volunteers to disease or infection. Since that course is impossible, the alternative is to look to the laboratory of the real world for more information. Over the years some researchers have used a deductive method of PNI research. That is, they studied sick people to find psychological features that preceded the disease or infection.

One of the first to concern himself with the association between mental states and physical health was Johns Hopkins' psychiatrist Adolph Meyer, who did his research shortly after the turn of the century. He was convinced that the occurrence of many of his patients' illnesses around the time they were experiencing some upheaval in their lives was not coincidental. Suspecting a connection, he asked his patients to supply certain information for a two-column "life record" form he designed. In the left column, Meyer noted the dates of the person's major illnesses; in the right column he listed important life events—moving to a new address, starting or finishing school, being fired from a job, and important births and death in the family—that occurred in those years. He used the chart for interviewing patients whom he labeled "psychoneurotic," individuals with vague physical symptoms having no easily discernible cause. Unlike many of his colleagues, Meyer believed that something medically important was occurring and deserved attention.

Out of his work came the suggestion that the occurrence of too many drastic changes in a person's life—a job change, pregnancy, the death of a parent—at one time may have physical as well as emotional effects. His approach systematized the collection of data related to the complicated emotional life of a patient. Although somewhat simplistic, it was the first step in the right direction.

Collecting this kind of information was refined even further in the mid-1960s by Navy psychiatrist Richard Rahe and University of Washington School of Medicine psychiatrist Dr. Thomas Holmes. Rahe had long been fascinated by the question of why some people become ill and others, living in the same place under the same circumstances, do not. His work was inspired by research in England in which doctors noted that among the patients they saw, those who were diagnosed as having tuberculosis had suffered noticeably more recent stressful life events than those who were disease-free.

In the early 1960s Holmes asked some tuberculosis patients to read over a list of common positive and negative life events and to indicate which events had happened to them. Then he asked a group of healthy people to do the same. When he compared lists, he noticed that the sick people had checked off more events.

At approximately the same time, Richard Rahe asked a group of sailors to check off a similar list before embarking on a six-month cruise. Over the next six months he kept close watch over the shipbound men. He found that those he called his high-stress sailors —men who had experienced more stressful life events—reported to sick bay most frequently with the most symptoms.

By the mid-1960s Holmes and Rahe combined their research efforts and tested more than five thousand individuals. After surveying thousands of people about how they would rate the various life stresses, Holmes and Rahe then distilled the number ratings into average estimates of the severity of each life stress. The result was the Holmes-Rahe Social Readjustment Rating Scale, a forty-three-item list of common experiences, which included minor events (such as taking a vacation) and emotionally devastating experiences (such as death of a spouse and divorce). To each they assigned a number rating according to its stress potency. (Death of a spouse rated 100, the highest; a minor violation of the law rated 11.) This was one of the first scientific measurements to consider *any* change, positive or negative, to be stressful and to emphasize that readjustment to an event is stressful.

The two researchers applied the scale to thousands of people: doctors, Navy personnel, heart attack patients, and medical students. Sifting through their findings, they concluded that the higher an individual's score rose over a total of 300 so-called life change units, the more likely it was that he or she would fall ill. Over the years the Holmes-Rahe scale, as it is more commonly called, has become a fixture in many stress studies (as well as a standard feature of magazine articles on stress).

The seductively simple scale (reproduced in Appendix A) offered an objective gauge for stress. But it has its limits. As Rahe pointed out, it can sketch the general outline of a person's experiences, but it does not take into account specific factors. Various circumstances, even an individual's personality, will affect the ways people react to events. To one person a vacation may be a welcome break from a year of hard work; to a workaholic it might be an annoying interruption and a source of dread. A widower living in a strange city far from family and friends may feel more lost than a widower living in his hometown surrounded by family and friends. A widow who was an abused wife might well view the death of her husband differently from a woman who has enjoyed a long and rewarding marriage. Individual circumstances and personal variables are difficult to rate.

Another variable is recall. Memories fade, sometimes rapidly. Over and over it has been confirmed that people asked to list significant events that have happened in the past year more than likely mentioned events of the preceding three to six months. Human memory is a frail and quirky facility. Except for extremely major events, most people's detailed grasp of the past extends only a few months back in time. Therefore, items on a list of life events may not be complete.

For all its limitations, the work of Holmes and Rahe was important in the exploration of the interrelationships between states of mind and states of the body. In search of those interrelationships a growing corps of PNI researchers has been studying the relation of the emotional jolts of life to the immune system. Some of the first clear evidence came, literally, from outer space.

During the *Apollo* flights in the 1960s and 1970s, NASA doctors noticed that the bodies of many astronauts experienced a shift in the number of their immune cells during reentry, one of the most stressful parts of the space mission. Over a two-year period, 1968 to 1970, NASA doctors studied the astronauts from the *Apollo VII* mission through the ill-fated *Apollo XIII* moon mission, the spaceflight that almost ended in disaster when an onboard explosion nearly marooned the crew permanently between the earth and the moon. On the day the men returned to earth, their lymphocyte (white blood cell) count was noticeably higher than on the day of liftoff.

NASA researchers then obtained similar findings with the three crews of *Skylab* astronauts who had spent one to three months in orbit. On splashdown day the potency of their immune systems was distinctly reduced. This finding was significant because tests on *Skylab* crews during the time they were in space found that their immune systems were low and that there was a surge in stress-related chemicals in their bloodstreams only on splashdown day.

With the NASA discovery came the first concrete evidence of stress as an immunosuppressant in humans. This research was especially interesting because the rugged astronaut corps was involved. All were carefully trained for the ordeal of space travel, were in excellent physical condition, and were veteran pilots who had experienced emergencies and crises in the sky. Even so, they were not immune to the trauma of space travel. (An especially interesting medical footnote to the *Apollo XIII* mission was that two of the three men developed respiratory infections during the flight.)

The NASA findings are fascinating, although they apply to a tiny percentage of the human race. However, at some time in their lives most people suffer the trauma of bereavement. In the laboratory of life the impact of the aftershock of grief on the operation of the immune system has been demonstrated. The first scientific suggestion of this impact appeared in 1969, when Dr. C. Murray Parkes, a British physician, and his colleagues at the Tavistock Institute of Human Relations in London published their study on widowers. They had carefully followed the health of 4,448 widowers, all fifty-five years or older, for nine years after the spouse's death. One of the most striking findings was that the widowers were dying at an unusually high rate within six months of their wives' deaths. Since many of these deaths were due to heart failure, the researchers called their study *Broken Heart*.

For years, medical folklore has held that bereavement is dangerous to one's health. Common sense accounts for some of the reasons: widows and widowers may overindulge in unhealthy habits—drinking and smoking more, using more tranquillizers or sleeping pills, eating less, not exercising—in general ignoring their health.

Looking beyond these commonsense explanations, a team of Australian researchers decided to study survivors' experience on a microscopic level. Dr. R. W. Bartrop and his colleagues administered a simple blood test to a group of twenty-six men and women who had lost their spouses. They took two sets of blood samples from this group: the first, two weeks after the spouse's death and the second, six weeks later. For comparison they also took blood samples from nonbereaved people of the same age and sex.

The two-week sample showed no detectable immune effect in either group, but at the six-week point the white blood cells of the widowers and widows were noticeably less responsive than those who were not grieving. It was a sign that their immunopotency had been diminished slightly in four weeks. This finding suggested that the aftershock of death required at least two weeks to produce a measurable effect on the immune system.

These results inspired other researchers to examine the bereavement effect more closely. At the Mount Sinai School of Medicine in New York, psychiatrist Dr. Steven Schleifer of the Department of Psychiatry had already been working in the general field of stress and immunity with his colleague, Dr. Marvin Stein. When he read about the Australian research, he decided to make a similar study, using periodic blood tests. Instead of following the survivors for a few weeks, Schleifer studied them for more than a year; since widowers typically were reported to have a higher mortality rate than that of widows, he concentrated his attention on the men.

Schleifer worked with a group of men whose wives were diagnosed as having terminal breast cancer; fifteen became widowers. Every month for a year after the spouse's death Schleifer took blood samples from the group and ran immunopotency tests on them. During the first two months after the death, their immune systems showed a sharp drop in responsiveness. Gradually their systems regained strength, but even as long as a year later, some men's immune systems had not rebounded completely. Although there was no absolute link between bereavement and the immune system, a cause-and-effect relationship is implied.

THE MINI-STRESS FACTOR

The average day does not include confrontations with death or major life stress, however. More often than not, it is a parade of less dramatic problems. Some are fixtures in a person's life (a chronically ill child, working with obnoxious associates), and others are random annoyances (delayed plane flights, sudden drenching showers). The overlooked annoying incidents also take their toll.

Sometimes they can overshadow the more dramatic pressures of life. Charles D. Spielberger, director of the University of South Florida's Center for Research in Community Psychology, and fellow psychologist Kenneth Grier were curious to find out which parts of police work were the most stressful. They talked to more than two hundred Florida police officers, asking them to rate the stressfulness of various aspects of their jobs. Duties such as "making arrests while alone" or "responding to a felony in progress" were rated much lower than "distorted or negative press reports" and were sometimes matched by "excessive paperwork."

Which mini-stresses are most annoying, of course, vary from occupation to occupation (in similar studies, teachers rated paperwork as a greater hassle) and from person to person, but the evidence remains that hassles should not be ignored. In findings reminiscent of those for Bourne's soldiers, University of Texas stress expert Robert Rose cites one study in which a group of firefighters showed no stress-hormone change during the high-pressure times of the work week but only on their days off.

That life should have this pattern is no surprise to psychologist Richard Lazarus of the University of California at Berkeley. It is his contention that although a scale or yardstick for measuring stress is useful, the measuring process presents problems. As insightful as Holmes and Rahe's scale is, it has drawbacks other than the ones already mentioned. One critical flaw cited by Lazarus is that no one checklist applies to everyone. Students, elderly adults, single parents, working mothers, and people with low incomes, to cite a few, face life stresses unique to their situations.

His second objection was that even where the scale is ideally suited to an individual, a high-risk score of more than 300, a supposed danger sign, does not guarantee illness. People have withstood more and have lived long, healthy lives. Third, he found the idea of focusing only on the changes in one's life a narrow approach. Times of change are stressful because they require adaptation. But what about situations that do not change but should? They might be equally stressful. What about the grinding, relentless pressure of a boring job or keeping oneself locked into a marriage that has gone sour?

Lazarus was among the first to wonder how much effect the so-called little problems have. "When someone is under pressure, petty problems that might otherwise be ignored—a broken shoelace, for example, can have a much greater effect than if they had occurred at less anxious times," Lazarus says. His work, therefore, has examined the way that such microcrises affect health.

To test his hypothesized hassle factor in health, Lazarus developed a checklist of 117 minor irritations and in one tryout run asked a group of one hundred Californians to match their lives against the list once a month for a year. He also asked them to keep track of more general psychological events: changes in moods, stress signals such as headaches or insomnia, changes or developments in physical health.

After sorting through the accumulated data, Lazarus found that hassles were better predictors of illness than major life events. This did not mean that there was no connection between a life crisis and illness. Indeed, those respondents who had experienced some major turmoil within two and a half years before they joined the Lazarus study seemed to be more susceptible to health problems, but his survey did show, on a month-by-month basis, that the hassle factor had a more immediate effect, especially among men. The more hassles they reported, the more negative emotions they felt and the more illnesses they reported. "In sum," Lazarus says, "it is not the large, dramatic events that make the difference, but what happens day in and day out, whether provoked by major events or not."

SURVIVALISMS

Whatever the source of the stress, a death in the family or a broken shoelace, why do some individuals manage to maneuver quite well the minefield of life? What factor makes a difference?

One factor of living that seems to be significant is social support: close emotional ties with friends or family. Although the apparent importance of such support seems intuitively correct, it is not readily susceptible to proof, because it is elusive, difficult to pinpoint, and even more difficult to document. Even to propose a way to support the hypothesis with evidence requires years of poring over a small mountain of information. One who tried is psychologist Lisa Berkman. While at the University of California at Berkeley in the mid-1970s, she found a study of seventy-three hundred Californians who had been interviewed about their life-styles and social relationships. Ten years had passed since the interviews were made, and Berkman was curious about what had happened to the people, seeing a good opportunity to test out the social support hypothesis.

Berkman grouped the people into those who lived lonely lives (no friends or relatives) and those who had rich resources of family and friends. Then she painstakingly examined the records of the state health department, cross-checking death certificates with the names of those surveyed. That done, she noted in which group the dead were included. Those she had classified as having had isolated lives were dying at three times the death rate of those with more social connections.

Obviously this is circumstantial evidence, but it does suggest a good connection between emotional closeness to people around you and length of life. But this connection was made after the fact. Psychologist James House and his colleagues decided to take a more direct approach, essentially watching people live for ten years. They persuaded twenty-seven hundred people in a small town in Michigan to participate in elaborate psychological interviews, after which they were rated according to a personal relationships scale, which noted items such as the number of a person's friends, degree of closeness to relatives, participation in group activities, and types of activities chosen. From the early 1970s to the early 1980s they studied the subjects; at the end of ten years the lonely had four times the mortality rate of those considered to be more social.

Probably the most detailed demonstration of a link between social groups and health was made by Dr. Leonard Syme, an epidemiologist at the School of Public Health at the University of California at Berkeley. He and his colleagues have spent years studying Japanese immigrants to the United States.

Japan is a country that both enjoys and endures all the good and bad features of life in the twentieth century. It is an extremely advanced, industrialized nation with many of the problems that accompany a high level of development. In and around the large cities, air pollution is horrendous, says Syme; smoking is widespread. The pace of life in their great urban centers is as frantic as in any Western city. Five-and-a-half- and six-day work weeks are still very common. Yet the Japanese have among the highest life expectancies in the world. Why?

Some researchers have postulated a genetic superiority among the Japanese, but that theory does not hold up very well. Within a generation of moving to the United States, Japanese immigrants who adopted our diets and life-styles succumbed to cancer and heart disease at the same rate as native-born Americans.

However, a sizable group is not so susceptible; some émigrés smoked heavily and consumed high-fat foods, all with impunity. Was there some factor that distinguished the healthy from the ill? After surveying approximately seventeen thousand Japanese, both in the United States and in Japan, Syme thinks that there is; the key, he suggests, is a certain characteristic of Japanese society.

Syme's indication of that characteristic came from the work of a colleague, Michael Marmot, who was studying groups of Japanese living in the San Francisco area. Marmot found that those Japanese immigrants who retained their cultural roots—used the language, socialized with other Japanese-Americans, and in general resisted Westernization—had lower incidences of heart disease and illnesses of all kinds. Other variables—genetic traits, age, sex, social class, even health habits—seemed to have little effect. The one common denominator that held true for the healthy group was they remained Japanese in spirit. That commitment to their group, and the support gained through it, kept them healthy, Syme believes.

Social support and social connections are extraordinarily important in that society. "To the Japanese, one's very identity is literally bound up with one's group," he offers. "One cannot think of oneself independently from the group. The importance of ties to others, to the community is the essence of Japanese culture and it is in dramatic contrast to western ways." In Japan an individual may spend a lifetime with the same group of people. He—this characteristic is most common among men—goes to school and is hired by the same firm, works, is promoted, and may be transferred with the same people. Breaking with so strong a tradition, says Syme, can literally be hazardous to one's health. "It seems most reasonable to conclude," he adds, "that interrupted social ties affect the body's defense system so that one becomes vulnerable, more susceptible to becoming ill from any one of a number of conditions."

Yet there may be times when a long-term disease creates a crisis, even in the best of families or among the tightest of social groups. Then the benefit of the support of others is limited. An example: George Washington University psychologist David Reiss did nine months of meticulous psychological and physical analysis of dialysis patients and followed their cases for three years, some until their death.

As the patients began to die, a pattern took shape; those who died tended to be the ones who came from very close, cohesive families, families notable for the way they conscientiously worked together to help one another solve problems. Yet the pattern of the high death rate of people with this background was so striking that even Dr. Reiss was nonplussed by his own discovery. The social support theory simply did not seem to apply. "We had thought the more accomplished, more cooperative families would have been a sustaining resource," he reported, "but they were more like the kiss of death."

Reiss had no clear explanation to offer, but one guess was that an illness in a family with a very strong group identity was more of a stress for the whole group than for a family not so tightly interconnected. Because the illness threatens the group, the patient may die so that the family can survive, he suggests.

Reiss's experience is a good object lesson in the pitfalls of rigid support of any one theory in PNI research. Life is seldom simple. At this time one can conclude that social support is a distinct and sometimes important so-called psychosocial factor that contributes to the manner in which an individual retains health and copes with illness. More often than not, it appears to be a positive factor, but, as David Reiss found out, it is not always beneficial.

THE SEARCH FOR HARDINESS

The larger question remains, why are some people survivors and others not? Suzanne Kobasa, psychologist at City University in New York, has spent her scientific career trying to find out. Since her graduate school days at the University of Chicago in the mid-

1970s she has been fascinated that some people who have experienced tremendous stress do not become ill. What do they have that the others do not?

The question came to mind when she was sitting in a doctor's waiting room, flipping through the pages of a magazine. Inside was an article on stress, including a find-your-stress-level test based on the Holmes-Rahe scale. The reader was supposed to check off applicable stresses and to determine the score. As Holmes and Rahe suggested, scores over 300 indicated that the reader was in danger of getting seriously ill. "Now my score was higher than 300, and I was still breathing. I was doing all right," she recalls. "So it seemed to me that wasn't the only way to interpret those results."

Several points bothered her about articles like the one she'd come across. One was that the hidden message of such articles is that people are often told to avoid stressful life events. But short of joining a cloistered order for the rest of one's life, it is impossible to avoid stress. "We might say no to a job promotion, but how do we say no to a parent becoming ill? It seems that the advice was somewhat limiting," she points out. "In the message avoid stressful life events was the idea that you should also walk away from positive events because they cause change and readjustment too. This struck me as both unrealistic and really limiting a person's opportunities."

A quality of stress that is often overlooked is that individuals need the challenge, the stimulation of stress in daily life. Some people forget that Hans Selye himself had a subspecies of stress he considered beneficial; he labeled it *eustress.* For some individuals it is a vitally necessary ingredient, the spice of life.

Individuals differ in the way they function under stress. Some people seek it and thrive on it (Selye called them racehorses), just as others seek out and require much less stimulation in their lives (Selye called these turtles). As if to underline this point, the Metropolitan Life Insurance company made an actuarial survey in 1974 of 1,078 men who held one of three high-level jobs in Fortune 500 companies. They may have been lonely at the top, but the stress did not abbreviate the executives' lifespans: The survey indicated that their mortality rate was more than a third lower than that of other white males of about the same age.

All too often the pop psychology in magazine articles advises avoiding stress at all costs. As psychologist Suzanne Kobasa likes to point out, many individuals can thrive on change and stress. People value new experiences, for that reason, they travel, or go on long camping trips, or take up new vocations.

Of course, some people can withstand more change and stress than others; Kobasa characterized such individuals as having *hardiness*. She describes this quality simply: "Hardiness should allow you to make the most of the situation."

For years Kobasa has been studying business executives, sorting out the healthy from the sick, the weak from the strong, trying to find out why one person effortlessly rides the waves of life while another sinks like a stone.

In a study of phone company executives in Illinois, she found her subjects divided actually into two distinct groups. Both were objectively considered to be under high stress. But only one group fell ill. The so-called hardy group had a much better health record. When Kobasa tried to determine the intangibles that might make the difference, she first examined such variables as their income, the religion they practiced or did not practice, and the prestige associated with their jobs. None of these factors seemed to matter. She then considered other possible explanations: that those who survived stresses were natural survivors because they had better genes; or that individual situations differed—the survivor group had more money, more support from their family, or other resources that produced different types of response.

One of the surprises of Kobasa's work was a discovery like David Reiss's, namely that having a supportive family and friends is not necessarily a guarantee of health. During her survey the phone company was going through the corporate trauma of divestiture, a chaotic situation creating a tremendous amount of pressure. She found that the unhealthiest executives, those who reported the greatest degree of stress and having the lowest "hardiness" rating, also claimed that they received a tremendous amount of support from their families.

To explain this anomaly, Kobasa suggests that only certain kinds of support from home or a friend tend to be beneficial. For example, in encouraging someone to complain but providing no help in working out solutions, a family is really offering little substantive help. "The family can become a kind of retreat," Kobasa says. The person who needs support gets the wrong message: "Instead of saying 'These people depend on me. They see me as a responsible person,' " Kobasa explains, "a person might say, 'They may not appreciate me at work but people love me at home.' "

Friendships, too, can work with or against a person. "There is a difference between using a friend's good wishes as a source of dependence versus using them as a way of reminding yourself that 'Yeah, I'm a capable person,' " she says. "Sometimes it's easier to use the support as an excuse and pull back from a stressful experience and go out for a pizza," adds Kobasa.

However, support is not irrelevant; some types of support have great impact. In another survey by Kobasa of respondents who said that they were under tremendous stress, those who felt they had the backing of their boss were ill half as often over the course of a year as those who said they received little support from their boss.

Far more significant than any kind of support are certain attitudes that typify the hardy individual. In sorting out the swimmers from the sinkers, says Kobasa, she found that the swimmers had a clear sense of who they were and what their values were. The key to this hardy personality was in the individual psychology of each person. After much more sifting and studying, she arrived at three trademarks of the survivors, traits sometimes glibly labeled the three C's: challenge, commitment, and control. The executives who did well felt stimulated by stress and change (challenge). They were intensely involved in what they were doing (commitment). And they usually did not feel powerless to affect a situation (control). Those who were not as healthy were without a compass. They had no sense of themselves or ways to adapt to change. "They told stories about having to come to work for the phone company ten years ago and now finding themselves in a totally different kind of environment. They talked about being tricked by the phone company in its new emerging form."

In Control

In the short history of modern PNI research, the importance of control recurs again and again. The two-rat experiment in which one animal simply lay there and received shocks whereas the other was able to control them provides a good metaphor for Kobasa's hypothesis.

In his learned helplessness experiments, psychologist Martin Seligman described the corrosion of willpower that comes with confronting an impossible situation over and over again. And while working with rats, Steven Maier showed how profound the effects of helplessness were: rats that could not control a stress also had depressed immune systems. Two Canadian psychologists, Lawrence Sklar and Hymie Anisman, took this work a step further by implanting cancer cells in two groups of mice. Each received identical electric shocks. One group could control the shocks and the other could not. The ones with no controls had faster growing tumors and shorter lifespans. The inability to cope with the stress, Sklar and Anisman say, was "tumorigenic," that is, it helped bring on neurochemical, hormonal, and immunological changes that made it easier for tumors to grow and flourish. Yet as is always the case with animal experiments, the question arises: do all these helpless mice and rats have anything to tell us about people?

One of the first to talk about control in humans was Dr. Arthur Schmale of the University of Rochester. He discussed the dark side of control, helplessness. He described the attitude as the "giving-up complex" and broke it down into individual components. Two elements were involved: *helplessness*, defined by Schmale as "a feeling of being deprived, let down or left out which was perceived as coming from a change in relationship about which the individual felt powerless to do anything," and *hopelessness*, a state of mind in which individuals are unable to meet their own standards, however unrealistic they may be.

When individuals lose some external source of gratification— through the death of a valued person, for example—a wave of helplessness/hopelessness may sweep over them. Individuals may feel that they are facing problems beyond their means. Schmale believes experiencing this complex of attitudes can lower individuals' resistance. As a result, they succumb to an illness or physical problem for which they are already disposed (asthma or arthritis, for example) or become ill or more ill. The giving-up complex does not cause disease, Schmale cautions, but disease frequently follows in its emotional wake.

This complex is not unusual or rare, according to Schmale. Everyone experiences it at one time or another, during some life transition. It happens as you lose or are giving up one person, goal, or identity and are adapting to that loss. It is part of the process of growing, developing, changing. For people who never learned to cope well, this giving-up complex can be volatile.

As an example, he cites the story of a woman leukemia patient being treated by one of his colleagues, Dr. William Greene. The disease was diagnosed shortly after the woman had been told that her husband, ill with tuberculosis, had little time left to live. The news was devastating. "When she first came to me she stated that she wanted to live until her son and only child, age 10 at the time, was grown up and settled," Greene recalled.

Over the years that followed, Greene noted the remissions and recurrences of her illness as measured by the changes in her blood cell count, an indicator of her body's efficiency in battling the disease. He noted, for example, that her blood count took a sudden jump at particular times of the year, just before his own annual summer vacation. He also noticed that her leukemia intensified during different crises in her life: during menopause and when she first acknowledged that her second marriage was failing. Her condition reached a critical stage when her son left home to go into the army. She deteriorated to the point that, for the first time in her life, she needed blood transfusions in order to stay alive.

The following four years when her son was in the military were very difficult for her. She was in and out of the hospital and was almost constantly undergoing treatments to keep the disease at bay. At the end of those grueling four years her son came home and announced that he was engaged to be married. Shortly afterward, she died, said Greene, as she predicted. Commenting on this case Greene wrote, "I suspect that the experience of most of us could attest to the likelihood that this occurs not infrequently."

These challenges to our sense of control are usually not so dramatic but people do confront similar problems almost daily. A situation exemplifying this point occurred while Kobasa was doing her research. The phone company was under pressure from the federal government to pay closer attention to affirmative action in its hiring, in other words, to add minorities to the payroll. The hardy executives reacted to the demand by saying something like, "I've got to change the makeup of my office, but how that's going to work is up to me." The unhealthy group simply saw the company memos on the subject as just "more memos coming down on *me.*"

One of Kobasa's more memorable subjects illustrating loss of control was an executive in his mid-thirties who visited her. He had decided to take her up on an offer she had made to the executives: that they could see their hardiness profiles. His psychological test showed his strong alienation: a disconnectedness from people and a lack of commitment to his job. (In fact, he later told Kobasa that he was leaving the phone company to start his own firm.) His medical history, for a man barely into middle age, was unusually dismal. He had most of the stress-related ailments: high blood pressure, peptic ulcer, migraine headaches. When Kobasa met him, she understood why.

The visit to her office, as she remembers it, was a catastrophe. The executive rushed into the office forty-five minutes late, commandeered her secretary's phone, and began making business calls to alert his cronies to where he would be. Kobasa recalls preparing to approach the sensitive topic of his apparent lack of connection to people. But she barely finished a sentence because each time her phone rang, the executive jumped up, convinced that the call was for him. The whole interview proceeded in this way.

"Finally he said to me, 'Look, I really need to take all these calls. They're very crucial. But you may have something here,'" Kobasa recalls him saying. "'So why don't you talk into my tape recorder' —and he pulls out a tape recorder and puts it on my desk— 'and I'll listen to it at night when I have a chance.' And he was probably the clearest case of someone I would call low hardiness."

This individual obviously was not a man in control. He could not shut the phones out of his attention for a moment; they ruled him. His deciding to leave the company underscored his lack of commitment, and his medical past was of a man who was not challenged by stress so much as brutalized by it.

To teach individuals to be flexible and adaptable in the face of stress, Kobasa has started what she calls a process of hardiness induction, basically a series of exercises for the stress-susceptible to teach them what they are doing wrong and to avoid self-defeating patterns of behavior. In one test of a group of executives, she found that after an eight-week session, there was a noticeable drop in the executives' blood pressure.

Kobasa's training begins with *focusing,* asking each person to zero in on some of the daily injuries and insults stress inflicts on the body. As an example, Kobasa says that she and her fellow researchers have noticed that many of the executives walk around with a day-long headache or knot in their stomachs. "They've always had this tightness in their stomachs or they've always started the day feeling a little queasy," she says. "It's kind of a new thing to think that well maybe it doesn't have to be there, to get them to see when they feel more tense, the times when the headaches seem to get worse or the knots in their stomachs seem to be more noticeable." This method indirectly causes people to recognize their feelings and the processes inside them.

The next step is to discover the phenomena that trigger that reaction and ways to handle it. Many people do not know at first what sets them off or misconstrue the cause. A headache or upset stomach is "not anger at the boss; it's really that they're frightened about losing their own job," she explains. This thinking through of cause and effect helps to shift the focus to where it belongs, gives them more insight into what is going on in their bodies, and enhances the "body sense," a self-conscious awareness of the effects of stress.

Another part of Kobasa's hardiness induction is asking people to pause in the course of the day to note how and when these pangs occur. She has found that taking the time to acknowledge the headache or stomach twinge is helpful.

To solve these problems, these individuals replay a stress situation in a process of *situational reconstruction*. Each goes back over a mishandled or traumatic situation at work, for example, and discusses it with the group. "Each person always thinks: 'it was miserable' and 'it turned out terrible for me'," Kobasa notes. "We have them think of how it might have been worse. People usually discover it wasn't as bad as it could have been." More importantly, they develop ideas for changing their behavior the next time and for avoiding repetition of mistakes.

Finally, the brutal fact is that for even the hardiest individual, life can be hard, and some problems are insoluble. Although she characterizes herself as a positive-thinking individual, Kobasa admits: "There are times when it is appropriate to say that life is miserable and no matter how hard you look for the silver lining, there may not be one. It would be a mistake to say if you smile and think good thoughts it's all going to be OK."

For those times when a problem does not recede despite a person's coping well, she recommends *compensatory self-improvement*: buttressing one's own damaged self-worth and self-esteem by shifting attention to something that one can control and that improves the quality of life. "There are things that happen that a person can't fix: like a child's being seriously ill or failing to save a doomed marriage," she says. "In the face of that kind of event, it may make sense to spend some time on another part of one's life where one can get positive feedback." For some people becoming involved in a new avocation or hobby, learning to sail, or taking lessons in a subject that interests them is effective. For others, concentrating on some part of their work that they can control or at least influence is beneficial. "Sometimes it's helpful to just pull back and let go and work on something else," Kobasa suggests.

However, sometimes we cannot pull back far enough, when the pressures around us touch us indelibly. We know from Bourne's soldiers, Maier's rats, and Schleifer's widowers what the general toll on the body can be, but how does the way individuals handle stress influence the way the body handles specific diseases?

CHAPTER SIX

Autoimmunity: The Body Against Itself

ON ALMOST ANY week of the year a group of men and women gathers in a room at Boston's Beth Israel Hospital to meditate. Different problems have sent them there: hypertension, heart disease, migraine headaches, diabetes, multiple sclerosis, or the excruciating pain of cancer. As part of their two-hour session the group sits on the floor and works at a self-directed mental exercise called *mindfulness meditation*. After a few minutes of concentrating on his breathing, a cancer patient, for example, focuses in on his pain. They are all there, as Joan Borysenko describes it, "to learn how to use their mind as a tool."

Borysenko is one of the developers of this program, officially known as the *Mind/Body Group*. The technique she uses is a variation of the relaxation response (see Appendix B for more information), the meditation method pioneered by Harvard cardiologist Dr. Herbert Benson. Borysenko is also one of the more innovative research-ers in PNI. Trained in both cell biology and psychology, she is an instructor at Harvard Medical School. Since the fall of 1981, she and her colleagues in the Mind/Body Group have been teaching people to marshall the powers of their minds to help themselves relax, to elicit the relaxation response, to learn how to change their own physiology, and ultimately to obtain "a sense of having control over themselves and control over their lives."

The Mind/Body Group is part of a program of the Division of Behavioral Medicine at Beth Israel Hospital headed by Dr. Herbert Benson. It is one of many programs being tried out around the country to help individuals suffering from a wide range of medical disorders, including arthritis and cancer.

Part of the goal of the program is to change attitudes. "What we really try to do is give people a sense of control over themselves and their lives. Many people are really unaware that they walk around depressed," she says. "What we are really trying to do is make people realize they are responsible for their own reactions; that they can learn to respond differently."

Patients like those of Joan Borysenko learn to exercise control to make their lives healthier and more enjoyable. In addition to the relaxation exercises, Mind/Body Group participants learn basics about nutrition. Those suffering from heart disease, for example, learn to take their own blood pressure. This program includes no drugs and no beliefs other than the patient's own conviction that the program will be beneficial.

Borysenko has been especially interested in the potential ben-efits of the relaxation techniques she teaches on a special group of patients: diabetics.

AUTOIMMUNE DISEASES: DIABETES

There are an estimated 6 million diabetics in the United States. These individuals have a greater risk of vision loss, kidney disease, strokes, and gangrene than the general population. It is the sixth most frequent cause of death in the United States and the second leading cause of blindness.

A diabetic's body cannot break down the sugars in the bloodstream and convert them to energy because of a deficiency in the hormone insulin, produced by the pancreas. There are two kinds of diabetes: type I and type II. Type I diabetes is treated with insulin injections. Type I diabetics usually develop the disease before the age of thirty and it is the most severe. Patients generally take insulin every day of their lives, and the gradual decay of the circulatory system characteristic of the disease is itself life-threatening. Type II diabetes occurs more often in later years, after age forty. Very often it can be treated by a careful diet, a habit of regular exercise, and medication to regulate blood sugar.

Over the years research results have suggested a psychological component to diabetes, especially to type I. Diabetes is one of a group of diseases called *autoimmune diseases,* a diverse group of disorders in which the immune system mistakes parts of its own body for the enemy. The hallmark of these disorders is inflammation varying from the merely irritating to the potentially deadly, as in diabetes.

The reasons that individuals contract diabetes are not clear. But a hereditary connection (the disease tends to run in families) has been demonstrated, and increasing evidence indicates that type I is an autoimmune disease, in which the immune system has damaged the body's insulin-producing capabilities. Researchers from Harvard Medical School and the Joslin Clinic in Boston, which specializes in diabetes research, believe that a defective immune system, specifically the system's T-cells, attacks and destroys the insulin-secreting cells in the body. Giving diabetics immunosuppressant drugs, still an experimental procedure, does seem to slow the progress of the disease.

It is known that the disease is stress-sensitive. (As long ago as 1679 one doctor suggested that "prolonged sorrow," that is, depression, was involved in the onset of diabetes.) Often considered a psychosomatic disease, diabetes has been studied by those seeking to isolate the psychological forces that influence it. Over thirty-five years ago researchers at Cornell University interviewed a small group of diabetics and found they could actually cause the balance of blood sugar in the diabetics' bodies to change simply by asking them to talk about stressful topics.

In the early 1970s psychiatrist Stefan Stein at Albert Einstein College of Medicine in New York did some tantalizing work suggesting that stress might also help activate diabetes. Stein wanted to know why diabetes mellitus strikes a particular individual at a particular time. For answers he looked to a nearby clinic, where he had been doing counseling work with adolescent diabetics. The hospital kept detailed records, including the age at which the youngster began to develop diabetes, and personal information about the family—how many divorces, separations, deaths, and family disturbances such as serious illness. Reviewing the records, Stein noticed that several teenagers were members of one-parent families. With the clinic's cooperation, Stein made a comparison study of diabetic and nondiabetic children of about the same age. He looked for family stability, "parental loss" (a parent missing because of death, divorce, or separation), and severe family disturbance: illness of both parents, a house in chaos, parental fighting. (He also had access to notes from pediatricians and social workers describing the family situations.) Finally, where such conditions existed, Stein was interested in whether they occurred before or after the onset of diabetes.

He found that well over two-thirds of the diabetic group had experienced parental loss or family disturbance; only a fifth of the other group showed similar circumstances. The real test of Stein's hypotheses was the time when the parental separation or the family problems occurred.

When he analyzed his results Stein found that in about half of the diabetes cases, some kind of parental loss had preceded the symptoms of diabetes. This finding suggested that a child born with a propensity toward diabetes could become diabetic as a result of a stressful family situation.

Stein's results did not prove a cause-and-effect relationship between stress and disease, but it suggested that psychological factors influenced the disease. The problem of quantifying the influence of psychological factors on diabetes remained.

Two Florida researchers, psychologist Margaret Linn and her surgeon-husband Bernard Linn, studied individuals afflicted with both kinds of diabetes to find out whether the insulin-dependent type I diabetics experienced stress differently from the type II diabetics.

The idea had been researched in studies of both humans and animals. In one experiment, psychologist Richard Surwit of Duke University found that when he stressed diabetic animals by immobilizing them in cages, their insulin levels dropped dramatically. In other tests, diabetic children injected with the stress chemical epinephrine also showed higher levels of blood sugar.

The Linns asked the diabetics to list some stressful events they had experienced recently and to rate the degree of stress they felt. Their questionnaires showed that those able to get along without insulin also had a sense of being less harried and pressured. The insulin-dependent group, by comparison, reported more stressful events in their lives, felt more stress, and felt it more intensely.

The researchers then administered a series of immune tests on both groups to look for any appreciable differences in immunopotency. On the whole, the insulin-independent group had relatively stable immune systems. The insulin-dependent group, on the other hand, registered an appreciably depressed immune system. The more the insulin-dependent group perceived themselves to be under stress, the lower was their immune potency.

The investigations into stress and diabetes have fine-tuned our knowledge of which diabetics appear to suffer the most from stress. They also underscored the power of disruptive life events to influence the course of the disease. At the same time they suggested a therapeutic approach—the relaxation exercises of Joan Borysenko, the biofeedback work of Richard Surwit—to counter the impact of the stresses. Work like theirs has taken medical therapy beyond gauging a diabetic's health by the amount of insulin in his body.

THE MIND–BODY APPROACH

One way of helping diabetics to cope with the potentially deleterious effects of stress is the program used by Joan Borysenko's Mind/Body Group. Except for a slightly greater emphasis on nutrition, her Mind/Body sessions for diabetics were identical to the ones she used with all her patients. However, her sessions are attended only by diabetics, creating a dynamic group identity that is therapeutic. The group members give each other social support in their relaxation procedures and encourage each other to follow the regimen.

Have Borysenko and her fellow Mind/Body researchers had good results? "We have," she says, "but I hasten to mention that it's a very small study. Our results are good in that those who practiced the Relaxation Response did have small changes in blood sugar. It was lowered." Changes have encouraged her to think about trying her technique on larger groups of diabetics. A drug-free assist in maintaining acceptable blood sugar levels could help minimize damage from the disease and help diabetics live longer, more trouble-free lives.

Biofeedback

Another body control method tried with some success on diabetics is biofeedback, used alone or with other relaxation techniques. The specifics vary, but the principle remains the same: *Biofeedback* is a technique that uses instruments to monitor certain bodily processes —muscle tension, skin surface temperature, brain wave activity, and pulse—and to mirror the activity they monitor. The way the mirroring is accomplished varies. Some instruments use a blinking light, and others use some sort of sound. The person whose body is connected to the biofeedback device can learn to modify body activities by listening to the tone or watching the light. The biofeedback method gives people using it a concrete measure of the degree of relaxation they are attaining. Individuals have managed to slow their heart rate, influence the amount of blood flowing to different parts of their body, and even change brain waves by responding to lights or sounds the biofeedback machine produces.

Biofeedback, used alone or with various other relaxation techniques, has helped individuals suffering from migraine headaches, hypertension, and an unusual ailment called Raynaud's disease (in which the arteries of the fingers and toes constrict during cold weather or sometimes during emotional upset; the spasms decrease circulation so much that the digits become pale and extremely cold and in severe cases develop ulcers or even gangrene at the tips).

Psychologist Richard Surwit at the Duke University Medical Center has used biofeedback to change the blood sugar levels in diabetics. Surwit says he managed to teach type II diabetics to raise the level of glucose tolerance in their bodies by biofeedback training. He chose a dozen diabetics whose disease was not sufficiently advanced as to require insulin but who did have difficulty maintaining their blood sugar levels in the safety range even with a special diet. Of the twelve patients, six received biofeedback and progressive relaxation training and six did not. Over a nine-day stretch in the hospital, the former group had one biofeedback session and three progressive relaxation exercises each day. By the end of the nine days, the six who did not receive the training were in essentially the same condition in which they arrived at the hospital, whereas the glucose tolerance of the six who had had relaxation training had improved noticeably.[1]

In another study, a twenty-year-old woman had recurring problems with hyperglycemia, a high level of sugar in the blood, whenever she felt stress. After six months of biofeedback training not only did her hyperglycemia attacks diminish, but her insulin needs dropped by half.

Controlling diabetes without drugs is a relatively new medical phenomenon—it does not offer anyone a cure, but an option unavailable until recently. Although the idea that diabetes can be treated from a PNI perspective is still fairly novel, the idea that autoimmune diseases might respond to this approach is not. One disease that figures prominently in the early history of psychoneuroimmunology is arthritis.

RHEUMATOID ARTHRITIS

In 1909, one doctor stated flatly, "That mental shocks, continuous anxiety and worry may determine the onset or provoke an exacerbation of rheumatoid arthritis is, I think, beyond question." In part because of its inclusion in the roster of psychosomatic diseases, rheumatoid arthritis has long been considered a disease with a powerful psychological component.

Like type I diabetes, rheumatoid arthritis is an autoimmune disease in which the immune system attacks the *collagen,* part of the connective tissue in the joint, causing inflammation. Of the diseases grouped under the umbrella of arthritis, rheumatoid arthritis is the most devastating. Unlike osteoarthritis, which affects people later in life, it strikes children as well as adults. (An estimated 250,000 children in the United States have juvenile rheumatoid arthritis.)

A simple blood test indicates the presence of a *rheumatoid factor,* a specific type of immunoglobulin (antibody) that is responsible for the attack. All individuals who have rheumatoid arthritis have this protein in their blood. But not all the people who have the protein contract the disease. Many have so-called arthritis autoantibody, which cancels the deleterious effect of the factor and provides immunity to the crippling disease.

Study after study has underscored the point that the psychology of an individual having rheumatoid arthritis can be an important feature of the disease process. For example, in the 1960s a team of doctors from the University of Rochester examined eight sets of identical twins, all women. Of each pair one twin was arthritic, the other, disease-free. In the course of their work the researchers uncovered a pattern in the way the disease appeared. The disease only seemed to surface after the arthritis sufferer had decided to expend her energies on dealing with a particularly stressful and distasteful situation. One woman, for example, decided to spend most of her life caring for her psychotic stepfather. Another woman took a job solely to impress her in-laws. In every pair the woman who became arthritic was the one who subjected herself to stress and seemed to seek it out. This discovery suggested that a characteristic of the psyche of the arthritic twin made her more disease-prone. Some element in her pattern of behavior and personality made her more susceptible.

To suggest that a type of personality could make one prone to arthritis would not surprise psychiatrist George Solomon, a pioneer in American PNI research. In the 1960s he and colleague Rudolf Moos, both of Stanford University's School of Medicine, were beginning their investigations into the medical myth that there were distinct rheumatoid arthritis personality traits. If this were true, Solomon wondered, how did those traits affect the development of the disease?

To address this question Solomon devised many clever experiments. One of the more ingenious was to study the behavior of a group of suspected arthritic patients. He used people who had come to the San Francisco General Hospital emergency room complaining of a tender, "hot," or inflamed joint. While the arthritic patients waited for laboratory test results, Solomon asked them to act out a brief psychodrama.

The theme of the psychodrama was the process of returning an item—a shaver for men, an iron for women—to someone playing a hostile department store clerk. Since a tendency to be unassertive and inhibited was hypothesized to be a distinct personality trait of arthritics, Solomon recognized in the situation a perfect opportunity to test the idea: here was a group of suspected, but as yet undiagnosed, arthritics in a role requiring assertiveness. Their participation in the psychodrama would allow Solomon to observe the hypothesized match between the personality and the disease.

After watching the psychodrama, Solomon made a selection among the participants. He found that he had identified all the individuals who later were shown to have rheumatoid arthritis through the inhibited and unassertive behavior with which they handled the drama in the returns department. Maybe the belief that some people had "arthritis personalities" had some validity.

Solomon's colleague Rudolph Moos reviewed everything that had been written on the arthritis personality and compiled a list of research reports of studies of over five thousand arthritics, designed to isolate some psychological constant among them. Evaluating the results, Moos concluded that the psychology of arthritis patients was distinctive: "The more closely one studies these patients," said one researcher, "the more [the] conviction grows . . . that the arthritic process is not merely frequently, but always, the expression of a personality conflict."

Moos and Solomon found evidence supporting the hypothesized personality traits of arthritics in comparing a group of arthritic women with their nonarthritic sisters. Aside from obvious personality traits, the arthritics seemed to be self-sacrificing, unable to express anger, and masochistic, sometimes to an extreme, in the way they lived their lives. One case Solomon recalls involved a woman who suffered years of abuse from her husband. The woman never complained. "You can't blame him; he had a mean father" was her explanation.

Solomon and Moos became convinced that distinct personality traits characterize individuals prone to most autoimmune diseases.[2] Generally, they are described as "quiet, introverted, reliable, conscientious, restricted in their expression of emotion, particularly anger, conforming, self-sacrificing, tending to allow themselves to be imposed upon, sensitive to criticism, distant, over-active and busy, stubborn, rigid, and controlling." (Curiously, he and Moos also found that many arthritics were notably athletic and sports-minded in their youth.)

A crisis of one kind or another or a shift in life-style could put the arthritic personality at risk. "The onset of disease," explains Solomon, "occurs either after a period of psychological stress, such as a loss of a significant person, or after the interruption of the ability to maintain a previously successful pattern of adaptation and defense. The professional athlete who, because of age, is forced to retire, for example, can't handle his aggression in that manner any more."

Because more people had the rheumatoid arthritis factor than had the disease, some special mechanism, some critical difference must distinguish the arthritis sufferers from those who are blessedly untouched. To find the element that made that difference, Solomon and Moos compared arthritics with nonarthritic relatives who had the same factor in their blood. They soon discovered that although the nonarthritic relatives had some of the same personality traits as the arthritics, their ability to cope seemed superior. "In other words, their personalities were similar, but the defenses were working," concludes Solomon. "Thus, in order to remain healthy, if one had this antibody which probably reflects genetic predisposition to rheumatoid disease, one had to be in good psychological condition as well."

To illustrate their point, Solomon and Moos compared a group of people who had the arthritis factor in their blood but did *not* have arthritis with a randomly collected group of people without the factor in their blood. The no-factor group generally reflected a representative cross section of humanity in their adjustment to life, "varying from really together to crazy—a bell-shaped curve," said Solomon. By comparison, the rheumatoid arthritis (RA) factor group were very healthy emotionally, extremely well adjusted. This result suggests that their superior coping ability may distinguish those who have the RA factor but do not have arthritis from those who do contract it.

Solomon suspects that psychological defenses are likely to be worn down by long-term stresses, such as the grueling ordeal of a bad marriage; for a person who has the masochistic traits of many arthritic sufferers, the combination of the long-term stress and the inability to give vent to one's frustrations—to express anger for example—could exacerbate the upsetting effects of a stressful situation. As the stress builds, the more likely is the body to succumb to the disease factor.

Of course, should a situation improve, the opposite result could occur. Solomon mentions one young patient, a woman who was on the verge of leaving her irresponsible husband, when she discovered that she was pregnant. During pregnancy, the woman's arthritic condition worsened, an unusual occurrence. Ordinarily pregnant women who have rheumatoid arthritis have relief from their disease, some suspect, because of changes in the immune system. "After the baby was born," Solomon reported, "her husband, who was delighted with the child, appeared to mature remarkably. The disease went into remission."

The mechanism by which a set of personality traits could set arthritis into motion is still one of the great unknowns in Solomon's theory. His general outline is that there is, first, a genetic predisposition to the disease. The body's submission to the disease factor may be accelerated by unknown physical reactions that accompany the inability to cope with the stress. In short, when individuals who have the RA factor leave the realm of the good copers and begin to feel the pressures of stress, their bodies reflect the strain by succumbing to the disease.

This hypothesis assumes that in the arthritic there is a mechanism through which the brain communicates with the body. Some researchers have proposed a psychoneuroimmunological link in the form of a distinct neurochemical. Rheumatologists at the University of California, San Francisco, and Massachusetts General Hospital have isolated a biochemical called *substance P* in the inflamed joints of arthritic animals. Substance P is a neurotransmitter: a chemical that signals a nerve to fire. It is a natural body product usually associated with the nervous system rather than the skeletal system. Yet the greater the degree of crippling, the more substance P arthritic animals had in their joints. Additional injections of substance P into the joint increased the severity of the arthritis.

Is a brain-body connection in arthritis possible? Although the evidence is still highly circumstantial, it is known that arthritics who have had strokes affecting one side of their body, for example, also suffer less virulent arthritis on that side. One of the obvious explanations is that the brain may be wired directly to the diseased area and that whatever occurs in the brain—attitudes, emotional reactions, responses to stress—is relayed over this hookup. Such a connection would constitute a relay system for the powers of the arthritic's personality and behavior.

Precisely what is being relayed over that system is still open to discussion. The idea of a personality specific to arthritis has not stood the test of time. Dr. George Solomon himself has qualified his earlier claim that there is a distinct arthritic personality. Revising his original hypothesis in the light of new evidence, Solomon now believes that the concept of disease-specific personalities is incorrect. "I have come to the tentative conclusion that there is not an 'autoimmune-prone,' 'cancer-prone,' or 'infection-prone' personality," he now concludes, "but rather there seems to be an 'immunosuppression-prone' pattern." He has broadened his definition of the personality to include ways of behaving and reacting to the world that might affect the style in which the body resists disease. Such moods and attitudes reverberate throughout the body.

Since Solomon and others first hypothesized an arthritic personality, research findings have explained some of the characteristics of the disease. For example, more women than men are victims. Solomon said this incidence in part reflects the effects of the submissive social roles women often assume, whether they want to or not. But neurologist Norman Geschwind of Harvard Medical School offered a more concrete explanation: that female hormones are involved in autoimmune diseases.

It is possible to explain part of the so-called arthritic personality trait of repressing feeling. A trio of researchers, Philip Spergel, George Ehrlich and Dorothea Glass at the Albert Einstein Medical Center in Philadelphia, made a personality match of arthritis sufferers and individuals having other chronic diseases. They found no personality differences between persons who had arthritis and those having other long-term diseases. No distinctive trait singled out the arthritics.

Yet they made another discovery. As a group, all the patients, arthritics and nonarthritics, had many common traits. Like the other patients, the arthritics were moderately depressed, "mildly hysterical," and prone to *somatization*, a tendency to let their emotional conflicts work themselves out through their bodies, via their particular ailments.

As a possible explanation for these results, University of Texas psychologist Jean Achterberg-Lawlis suggests that alexithymia, the inability to verbalize emotions, could account for the unemotional manner of some arthritics. According to the theory, this emotional flatness is not the result of any personality disorder but of a poor neuronal link between the two halves of the brain. The right, emotional side of the brain cannot find expression through the verbal left side of the brain because of poor communication of emotional information across the two sides of the brain. As a substitute for expressing emotions verbally, a person might do so physically, through illness.

It is also possible that the disease precedes the personality traits. Achterberg-Lawlis points to one comparison study of newly diagnosed arthritis patients, patients with other chronic diseases, and patients who had been suffering from rheumatoid arthritis for a long time. The only groups that resembled each other in personality were the newly diagnosed arthritics and those who had had the disease for a long time. This finding, she said, could be explained one of two ways. Either an arthritis personality might have been manifesting itself, or the painful and crippling effects of the disease shaped the behavior and attitudes of the victims. Rather than the personality causing the disease, the disease might have produced a distinct personality. Perhaps George Solomon's arthritic personality traits were merely the consequence of living with a chronic disease.

Implicating stress as part of the arthritis disease process may lead to oversimplifying psychological factors. As was mentioned earlier, psychiatrist Malcolm Rogers and his colleagues at Harvard Medical School challenged this assumption by attempting to induce arthritis with a combination of chemicals and stress in a group of rats. In trying this combination, Rogers had curiously mixed results. In one experiment he crowded a group of genetically identical rats injected with arthritis-inducing chemicals into a small cage while a large cat lurked outside.

On comparing the terrified animals to a group that spent the duration of the experiment resting cat-free in other cages, Rogers found that over a third of the nonstressed rats developed arthritis, whereas only one of the stressed animals did. In a later experiment he substituted 100-decibel blasts of noise as the stressor. This time the result was much different. More of the stressed rats succumbed to arthritis than those that had had peace and quiet. This result suggested to Rogers that arthritis is affected by stress, but the effects may surface in different ways; in the words of his studies, they might be modulated by the stress. Some stresses, such as the noise, could exacerbate the condition. Others, such as the cat, could help keep the disease in check. Also, the animals got different stresses at different times of the day—a significant fact since the immune system has a circadian rhythm. Its strength varies over a 24-hour period.

The experience has left Rogers convinced that arthritis is susceptible to psychological influences induced by stress. But the mystery is that the influence is not always in one direction, as the experience of his predator-frightened and noise-stressed rats testify. Less durable is the idea of a personality specific to arthritis; that concept has not held up consistently over time. Yet it is an idea that proved to be of tremendous value in the history of PNI. Studying personality traits and arthritis shifted the focus of medical attention from the purely physical to include the psychological as well. In its early forms, particularly the work of Solomon and Moos, the study of personality factors broadened the breadth and depth of medical interest in behavioral factors and disease.

Arthritis Therapies

A few behavioral programs for arthritis have been created, the partial result of insights gleaned from early PNI research. Currently, there are only a few therapies, recommended for alleviating some of the suffering caused by the disease. One is exercise, whose chief benefit is to move the blood flow to the affected joints and to keep them flexible. Typically, arthritic patients do stretching exercises to ensure that the joints move smoothly and do strengthening exercises to maintain muscle tone. Also recommended are exercises for general fitness and flexibility. Walking and non-weight-bearing exercises such as swimming are particularly beneficial.

Lately, individuals working in the field of arthritis have been trying another method. At the Stanford University Arthritis Center, doctors use relaxation tapes for their patients; these tapes can be purchased from the sources listed in Appendix C. The logic for using the tapes is simple. If the mind is distracted by mental exercises, it is not feeling the pain of the arthritis attack. At the very least, this method alleviates stress and discomfort. In addition, some experimenters believe that the relaxation response increases the body's production of natural painkillers, endorphins. If this is true, relaxation could have an analgesic effect as well.

Using a similar approach, psychologist Jean Achterberg-Lawlis has obtained encouraging results through a program of pain and stress management that uses biofeedback to train people to relax. In one experimental therapy, a group of arthritic individuals diminished the amount of pain they were feeling, reduced the tension created by the pain, and in general slept better. In another, one group of arthritics had biofeedback training and another had a standard physical therapy program. Not only did the group employing biofeedback and relaxation feel better, but an erythrocyte sedimentation rate (ESR) blood test measuring the activity of the disease showed that the immune system had held stable against the disease or the arthritis had abated.

Similar programs using mind exercises such as progressive relaxation have also had encouraging results. Achterberg-Lawlis is not certain why they are effective but proposes a possible explanation. Relaxing exercises primarily reduce muscle tension, thereby decreasing sympathetic nervous system activity. A less active nervous system may make life easier for the arthritis sufferer, especially since the discovery of substance P in arthritic joints. When fewer signals are sent to the stricken areas of the body, less irritation of the stricken joints may result.

The strong undercurrent of psychological forces that has existed in autoimmune diseases suggests that individuals having those diseases may benefit from exploring the effects of these personality and behavior patterns. Psychotherapy has often been useful in helping patients understand the emotions underlying their symptoms. Using self-soothing techniques—relaxation exercises, mindfulness meditation, biofeedback—are another way to detoxify disease-enhancing behavior in autoimmune diseases. These strategies involve the mind in a conscious role in a situation in which it may already play an unwitting role.

CHAPTER SEVEN

Out of Control

ONE OF THE more wonderful of medical stories is one told by a nineteenth-century Baltimore physician, Dr. John Noland MacKenzie, entitled "The Production of the So-called 'Rose Cold' by Means of an Artificial Rose." The story involves one of his patients, a woman "thirty-two years of age, in excellent circumstances, surrounded by all the comforts of life; very stout, well nourished, but physically weak; five feet high, with light brown hair, brown eyes, and fair complexion," and, the doctor added, "nervous temperament."[1]

Every year, for fifteen years, from May until September, the woman suffered from violent coryza (runny nose), and severe asthma attacks, especially in the latter part of the summer. "During the attack the temperature ranges between 100°F and 105°F." These

attacks were so violent that the woman sometimes lapsed into unconsciousness.

Almost any stimulus could provoke the attacks. MacKenzie
listed seventeen items from fright, overexertion, and sudden excitement, to exposure to "night air." She seemed especially sensitive to
the odor of hay and roses. "Last summer, while on a visit to the
country," MacKenzie wrote, "she was immediately seized with
coryza; and on several occasions while passing a haycart in the
thoroughfares of the city was taken with an attack of asthma." He
summed up: "She has tried almost everything known to the profession and laity, including a host of quack specifics, for the relief of
her trouble, but without making an impression on her disease."

After observing and treating her for a few days, the good doctor
had a plan. "Decidedly skeptical as to the power of pollen to produce a paroxysm in her particular case, I practised the following
deception upon her, which still further confirmed me in that belief,"
he wrote. "For the purpose of the experiment, I obtained an artificial
rose of such exquisite workmanship that it presented a perfect
counterfeit of the original."

During her next visit, the woman was telling the doctor how
much better she was feeling when he began his experiment. "I
produced the artificial rose from behind a screen where it had been
secreted, and, sitting before her, held it in my hand. In the course
of a minute she said she felt she must sneeze." Within five minutes
the woman was having a full-fledged allergic attack, exactly what
she would be suffering if the doctor had been holding a real rose.
"When I told her that the rose was an artificial one, her amazement
was great, and her incredulity on the subject was only removed
upon personal examination of the counterfeit flower," MacKenzie
noted. "She left my office with severe coryza, but also with the
assurance that her disease was not altogether irremediable." A few
days later, the woman returned to the doctor's office and "on that
occasion she buried her nostrils in a large fragrant specimen of the
genuine article and inhaled its pollen" with not so much as a sneeze.

This is an example from the annals of medicine of as pure
a psychosomatic ailment as you are likely to find. Today many
would say that the cause of the woman's rose cold lay not in her
nose, but in her head. In the past fifteen to twenty years, volumes of research papers have been published on "psychogenic
factors," "psychic factors," "personality correlates," "psychological

dimensions," "psychological aspects," "personality traits," "life-style factors," "behavioral-physiological factors," and "behavioral and social contributors to disease." Out of a blizzard of research reports, despite their uneven quality, one conclusion keeps surfacing, that mental states can be medically important in almost every disease, including allergies and even infectious diseases.

ALLERGIES: ASTHMA

The belief that psychological forces may trigger a specific disease has long prevailed for many diseases. One of the first with which this belief was associated is asthma; Hippocrates warned asthmatics to "guard themselves against anger" to avoid their debilitating attacks.

Described simply, *asthma* is an allergic condition in which the body reacts to allergens by contracting the breathing tubes of the lungs, the bronchi and bronchioles, provoking a range of respiratory problems from mildly annoying wheezing to total closure of the breathing tubes, asphyxiation, and death.

Observing a severe asthmatic attack is frightening; experiencing one is terrifying. The attack is provoked when an asthmatic inhales an allergenic substance or feels certain strong emotions; even crying and laughing may trigger it. Within the body the muscles around the lungs' bronchioles or smaller breathing tubes go into spasm, preventing the asthmatic from exhaling. More often than not, a person panics at being unable to breathe out. That panic makes the tubes constrict more, and the vicious cycle continues until the attack passes, the asthmatic uses medication to open the tubes, or deposits of mucus form, suffocating the asthmatic to death.

The immune system is intimately involved in asthma attacks; the cause is an overreaction to the antigen. Asthma sufferers carry around in their genes the trait of overreacting. In many cases, emotional factors exacerbate the virulence of an attack. Asthma typically afflicts boys slightly more often than girls, but by adulthood the incidence is equal for both sexes.

One of the mysteries of the disease is that there is no consistent pattern to its intensity or frequency (some people even "grow out" of asthma on passing from childhood to adulthood). According to Thomas Creer, an Ohio University psychologist who specializes in studying the disease, no two patients have the same intensity of attacks. One may feel only a little breathing discomfort, while another will feel as if he is about to suffocate to death. Also a patient might have different patterns of attacks, having no problems for months and then enduring a spell of attacks that appear with a baffling suddenness. The disease is highly variable.

The reason for this variability, suggested psychiatrist Franz Alexander, considered a founder of modern psychosomatic medicine, is the *summation of stimuli:* sometimes an asthma attack can occur only when both an allergic factor and an emotional stimulus are present.

Alexander favored a decidedly psychoanalytic approach to asthma. He did not believe that there is a typical asthmatic personality: "we find among persons suffering from asthma many types of personalities: aggressive, ambitious, argumentative persons, daredevils, and also hypersensitive, aesthetic types. . . . It would be futile to define a characteristic profile; no such profile exists." But Alexander did believe that the asthmatic's background provided a psychological clue: "The repressed dependence upon the mother is, however, a constant feature around which different types of character defenses may develop," he said.

Alexander's portrait of the asthmatic is heavy with Freudian psychoanalytic overtones. Anything that competes for the mother's attention can provoke an attack, he suggested. Children may begin to have attacks following the birth of a new brother or sister who may draw off the mother's affection. For adults an attack may occur when they face sexual temptation or even marriage, a threat to the relationship with the mother. For them, the asthma attack is a suppressed cry for the mother. (One of literature's more famous asthmatics, Marcel Proust, often wrote of suffering severe asthma attacks after having violent arguments with his mother.) Alexander felt that since the disease is freighted with so much meaning, psychoanalysis offers help in alleviating the symptoms. Followers of Alexander have even gone so far as to postulate an asthmatic personality.

"That theory had quite an impact and hung around for a long time," admits Dr. Peter Knapp, a Boston University psychoanalyst who has made the disease his life's study. "And one does see cases where it does apply. But I think most people who work with asthma now feel even that version of the personality theory is too general to be useful." Thomas Creer agrees that the idea has not stood the test of close analysis. Families of asthmatic children have been interviewed, run through battery after battery of tests, observed in the home, and on the whole nothing aberrant or abnormal showed up in the children's relationships with their mothers.

There may indeed be a pattern of behavior, but it is very hard to sort out which personality traits predated the asthma and which were the result of this episodic, potentially life-threatening disease. Investigators have variously characterized asthmatics as being depressed, hostile, anxious, defiant, introverted, intelligent but inhibited, covertly aggressive, and dependent.

Given all this confusion, Thomas Creer says that there are "simply no data to support the contention that there is a unique personality characteristic of those with asthma." Peter Knapp agrees up to a point but claims there are psychological factors asthmatics have in common, and dependency is one. Here one runs into a chicken-or-the-egg problem. "If a person has a life-threatening disease, they're apt to be dependent—on the medication, on whoever supplies it."

"The trouble with asthma," he continues, "is [that] it is a slippery disease. The actual cause of the disease is not always that clear and there are different kinds—adult asthma, and childhood asthma, which is quite a different beast. And there is a miscellaneous collection of other subtypes which we don't know much about."

These statements do not exclude the possibility that psychological components are present. Almost thirty years ago, a doctor conducted some clever experiments with a group of children who were genuinely allergic to the dust in their homes. When they were asked to inhale air sprinkled with house dust, the children quickly developed asthma attacks. After the children were taken to a hospital, the experimenters took dust from each child's home and sprayed it into each hospital room. Away from the cues and familiar surroundings of the home, nineteen of the twenty children had no reaction.

Conditioning is a powerful element in disease, one that has more than superficial effects. As a demonstration of that power, experimenters Michael Russell and his colleagues at the Brain-

Behavior Research Center of UCLA injected a minute amount of foreign animal protein, BSA, into the footpad of some guinea pigs and allowed their systems a chance to develop the expected allergy. A month later, the animals were made to sniff a cotton swab tinged with a noxious sulfurous smell and the allergy-causing animal protein. Blood samples from the animals showed that their bodies released the allergy chemical histamine in reaction to the protein.

Later Russell and his team gave the animals cotton drenched with the same foul-smelling sulfur but without the antigen. Blood tests again showed that the animals' bodies reacted with a jolt of histamine, as though they were still exposed to the antigen. The guinea pig test, Russell says, showed that nonphysiological elements, such as cues from the environment (in this instance, the sulfur smell) can trigger an allergic response. This process of associative learning, as he called it, is an important and often overlooked element in many animal and human allergies. Some individuals respond as the guinea pigs did, with allergic reactions, for no discernible reason. "They keep being told that it's psychosomatic, or that they're crazy," says Russell, "but in many instances it is behavioral conditioning."

Equally ingenious experiments have shown the power of behavioral conditioning on people. One of the best examples was performed by a group of Dutch physicians in the late 1950s. They had heard the story of Dr. MacKenzie's patient and her reaction to the artificial rose and of a man so allergic to horses that an attack resulted even when he saw horses in a movie. For their experiments, the Dutch team asked some asthmatics to enter their laboratory and act as their guinea pigs.

The people sat down before a wooden box. Snaking from it, in a hookahlike arrangement, was a series of rubber tubes with a glass straw or mouthpiece at the breathing end. From the asthmatic's seat, the tubes' connections were invisible. Each day for a few minutes the asthma patients sat and breathed through the rubber tubes. On some days they were breathing an allergy cocktail, oxygen laced with grass pollen or house dust, on others a mist of plain saltwater and baking soda. By carefully orchestrating the order in which an asthmatic breathed these different substances, the experimenters were able to produce conditioned responses of asthma attacks.

One of their more spectacular cases was a thirty-seven-year-old unmarried woman who went to the laboratory in Amsterdam, sat in front of the box with the rubber tubes, and breathed through them for twenty minutes every few days for about a month. In the beginning she breathed the harmless neutral mist first and then the allergic solution. At first nothing happened, but when she began breathing the pollen-rich mist, not surprisingly, she experienced a violent asthma attack. In the following sessions the experimenters switched the order in which she breathed the substances, administering the pollinated mist first each time. Again she reacted only when she breathed in the allergenic mist.

That procedure was followed by another switch. The experimenters returned to their first pattern (saltwater mist first; allergen, second). When the woman breathed in the innocuous mist, "to our amazement, the patient reacted with subjective and objective dyspnoea [gasping] and wheezing during inhalation," the team reported. Thinking some of the allergic substances were still in the tubes, the scientists installed new breathing tubes.

They asked the woman to return five days later to try again. When she returned, they gave her pure oxygen to breathe. She had another asthma attack. Thinking she might have developed an allergy to the rubber breathing tubes, they replaced them with plastic ones. The woman tried again, having another asthma attack. The experimenters used a new mouthpiece made of glass; she had another asthma attack. Suspecting that there might even yet be some infinitessimal amount of some allergic substance in the oxygen she was breathing, they asked her to sit with the new glass mouthpiece between her lips and simply inhale the air in the room. Within five minutes, another asthma attack began. They took her to a different room and asked her to breathe through the tube: another asthma attack: "the patient had now reached a state where it was possible to provoke an attack of asthma within a few minutes by simply asking her to hold a piece of glass in her mouth," the doctors reported. They had instilled in her a conditioned, or learned, response that was so deep that the presence of any allergic element was irrelevant to the attack.

If conditioning is a powerful component in asthma, strong emotional crises may also be. "Just the other day a doctor called to discuss one of his patients, a woman in her forties with very very severe asthma," recalled Boston University's Dr. Knapp.

She's in and out of the emergency ward every other month. Her husband died of leukemia eighteen months ago and son committed suicide two years ago. She's had this severe asthma ever since.

I've seen maybe a couple of hundred asthmatics of varying intensity over the years and that is such a familiar story to me: late onset, depressive coloring, something very major in life precipitating it. If you saw the patient, her depression would be very muted and you'd be hearing about her terrible symptoms.

As in many other diseases, the cause of asthma is complex. There is a powerful genetic element to the disease: between 40 and 75 percent of asthmatics have the disease in their family histories. But other elements are also at work. Although there is no distinct asthmatic personality, many sufferers share certain traits: depression, lack of assertiveness, low self-esteem, and inability to make social contacts.

Knapp studied brothers, identical twins, with family histories of asthma. One suffered from mild depression and began having periodic asthma attacks within months of a traumatic separation from his family, being hospitalized for scarlet fever. His brother, more easygoing, also had similar asthmatic tendencies, but except for an occasional bout of hay fever and one attack of "baker's asthma," the result of working around the irritating dust in a flour factory, he was trouble-free. The difference between the two cases, says Knapp, was that one boy was more vulnerable to emotional asthma triggers.

As an explanation of these different responses, Knapp proposes an additive hypothesis: that both psychological and biologic factors influence the outcome of the disease so "that their combined strength determines the severity of the final disorder."

Treatments

Asthma has no cure, and, for the moment, no single recommended method of treatment. Various techniques have been tried, according to Dr. Knapp, including antianxiety medication (tension and anxiety may cause asthmatics to hyperventilate); behavioral techniques such as transcendental meditation, biofeedback, and hypnosis; and various kinds of therapy: group therapy, family therapy, and long-term psychotherapy.

The results of using these techniques have been interesting but mixed. Antianxiety drugs do help some people, but the numbers appear to be small. Some behavioral techniques also seem to help: asthmatics who practiced transcendental meditation for three months did show a dramatic improvement in their conditions, as did children who tried biofeedback devices, machines that measured the muscle tension in their faces. After a little training, they learned to relax the fine muscles in their faces and to improve their breathing as well.

Knapp's own suggested approach has two components. First is treating the medical symptoms of the asthmatic individual with whatever drugs are suitable. Second, Knapp recommends trying a "meta analysis" approach, using the techniques of family therapy, group therapy, individual therapy—whichever is appropriate. Using therapy requires a longer-term commitment by the therapist, says Knapp, because the "somatic and psychic difficulties" of an asthmatic are, as he puts it, "extraordinarily intertwined."

Psychotherapy may be useful, says Creer, but behavioral conditioning that helps break some of the behavioral hold asthma has over those afflicted with it seems to be more effective. He has initiated techniques as basic as teaching patients, especially children, what a true asthma attack is like to help them avoid the constant state of panic or dis-ease that may characterize the life of an asthmatic. Creer has developed so-called attack behaviors, techniques for minimizing the intensity of the asthma attacks and the period of hospitalization required for recovery. One simple method is requiring that asthmatics spend a part of each day talking to other patients to remove them from their self-involved role as professional patients. The individuals who practiced this technique entered the hospital half as often as they had previously and stayed for much shorter spans of time. A final objective measure of improvement, Creer says, is that the patients needed less medication than they had before.

INFECTIOUS DISEASE

Some of the most dramatic evidence that the mind-body factor is a real element in health has come from research with infectious diseases. In infectious diseases a simple cause-and-effect relationship should prevail. An infecting microbe (cause) attacks a target (the body), producing disease (effect). But the phenomenon is not so simple. Why is it, if you expose a randomly selected group of people to a germ, that everyone does not become ill?

Obviously, to contract a disease a person must be susceptible. But that susceptibility does not explain the difference. For example, some experimenters tried to infect some volunteers with streptococcus bacteria, as universal an infectious agent as one is likely to find. But as few as one-fifth of those exposed to the streptococci contracted the infection. Somehow the remaining four-fifths were protected.

Some of the early work done to solve this mystery involved respiratory ailments, initially tuberculosis. As writer Susan Sontag points out in *Illness As Metaphor,* a specific state of mind is associated with TB. It has to be one of the few diseases whose victims have been the subject of romantic lore, from Thomas Mann's comfortably suffering Hans Castorp in *The Magic Mountain* (inspired by his own wife's stay in a mountain sanitorium) to the tragic Lady of the Camellias in *La Traviata.* The classic TB victim was sensitive, alternately mournful and passionate. Some individuals were considered to be tuberculosis-prone by reason of their temperament, in a sense doomed by their creativity and sensitivity. Tuberculosis was the disease of artists.

The reality of the disease was different. Before cures and controls were found, tuberculosis was a leading killer in the late nineteenth and early twentieth centuries, known as the Great White Plague, according to René Dubos. The actuarial data indicate that about one in one thousand people stood a better than average chance of contracting TB. The disease is treacherous: it fluctuates over time, flaring up one month and leaving a victim symptom-free for years. Why does the disease attack some and leave others barely touched by infection?

In a landmark survey of the way life events affect illness, Judith Rabkin and Elmer Streuning, two researchers from the Epidemiology of Mental Disorders Research Unit of the New York State

Department of Health in New York City, reviewed more than seventy studies relating disease to upheaval in society and in individual lives.[2] Two of the studies examined tuberculosis, correlating the disease with disruptions associated with relocating to a new home or new land. One survey pointed out that the Irish who emigrated to New York during the great famine of the 1800s were materially better off than those who stayed behind. Nevertheless, their death rate from tuberculosis was much higher than that of their poorer Irish relatives: the tuberculosis death rate among the Irish in New York was twice that of Dublin. Another group of researchers discovered that when a group of American Navajo were moved from their homeland to a new reservation, a sudden and "appalling" increase in the death rate from tuberculosis resulted, even though the new reservation was only a few miles away from the old one.

Rabkin and Streuning wrote what was for its time (the mid-1970s), the ultimate survey on the ways that social conditions affect a person's susceptibility to disease. For example, people who live an unstable, transient life are statistically more prone to illness, as are members of a *low-status minority* (recent immigrants to an area). An individual caught in a *status inconsistency*, for example, a person over-qualified for his or her job, also has a higher than average incidence of illness: a Ph.D. in anthropology who drives a bread truck or someone who has been promoted to a new social and economic level (a blue-collar worker who steps into a white-collar manager's position). And as mentioned previously, changes in the social environment, such as the culture shock of immigration, also seem to increase susceptibility to illness.

These conclusions were all reached through statistics—disease rates, population size—not specific medical cases. In theory disruptions and upset appeared to influence disease susceptibility. One of the more exhaustive modern studies of infectious disease and stress was an experiment involving the common infectious disease mononucleosis; the subjects were a new class of cadets at the U.S. Military Academy. For four years Yale University researcher Stanislav Kasl studied the pattern of mononucleosis infection among the cadet class; his findings demonstrated the interaction of psychosocial factors and "germ theory."

Using a simple blood test, Kasl and his research group found that of the 1,400 cadets, 432 were "susceptibles," cadets not immune to mononucleosis. Over the four years, 97 of the 432 dropped out of the academy; 141 went through all four years with no infection; and one group, 194, contracted mononucleosis at one point or another during their four-year stint at the academy. How, Kasl wanted to know, were those 194 different from the others?

He had two sets of information to work from: medical data, including that first blood test and reports of all visits to the academy infirmary, and an amalgam of psychological information for each cadet—results of psychological tests given during the enrollment process, four-year academic records, and family information.

Sifting through all this information, Kasl found three common denominators for the ill cadets: Their fathers were described as "overachievers" (their accomplishments exceeded their educational or sociological background); the cadets themselves were deeply committed to following a military career; finally, these same young men performed poorly academically. An added bit of information was that the lower the academic rating of people in this infectious group, the more likely they were to have a severe case of mononucleosis.

Kasl's four-year disease watch showed the complexity a straightforward case of simple infection could present. Many ingredients seemed to be at work in making individuals candidates for the disease, most obviously, a susceptibility to it. Kasl uncovered the three psychosocial elements in his cadets. Also important was the interplay of the three factors in swaying the defensive powers of the immune system. For example, wanting a military career badly was a riskier attitude if the student performed poorly scholastically. Those who had the volatile combination of poor grades and a strong desire to be a career officer contracted the disease most frequently and stayed longest in the hospital. Conversely, as the cadets' grades improved or their commitment to a military career diminished, they either did not become sick or, when they did, were not incapacitated for very long.

The connection between respiratory problems and psychological influences has been well documented. One particularly ingenious study that tried to match personality with disease susceptibility was conducted by Harvard University psychologist David McClelland and former colleague John Jemmott. McClelland says that a certain kind of person has a high need for power. Such a person also has what McClelland calls a low need for affiliation, meaning little interest in close relationships of family and friends. Finally, this individual has a tremendous amount of self-control, in extreme cases, suppressed hostility. In the business world, McClelland says, this type of person is an adept manager of people and an empire builder.

He devised a simple interview test to sort out these individuals and over the years has focused on them in his research. When these people are under stress, that is, feel their need for power frustrated, their bodies secrete high levels of epinephrine and norepinephrine, both chemicals he believes to be associated with diminished immune powers.

To test his hypothesis, McClelland and Jemmott sorted out a group of dental students according to whether they could be rated as high in the need for power and followed the students over the year. Those rated as high in *inhibited power motivation,* as the profile came to be called, had more colds during the year, usually around exam time, than did those low in inhibited power motivation.

Although the common cold is a good litmus test for susceptibility, almost everyone contracts one every year. In fact, the idea that even the common cold had a psychological element so intrigued pediatricians Roger Meyer and Robert Haggerty that they decided to test for an even more common germ, streptococcus bacteria, commonly present in children. Certain virulent streptococcus germs cause sore throat, ear infection, or scarlet fever. Just as importantly, the streptococcus they chose was usually benign. "Peaceful coexistence between this organism and its human host is the rule, while disease is the exception," Meyer and Haggerty noted.[3] Many children harbored the bacteria, but only a fraction of them became ill because of it. Meyer and Haggerty hoped to find out why.

They watched sixteen families, with two or more children each, for a year. Every three weeks the two doctors checked on the family's health and took throat cultures from everyone. The results were compared against a shopping list of factors: the child's age, sex, family health history, antibody response, whether the child had had a tonsillectomy, housing (number of rooms at home and type of heating system), size of the family, special stresses at home, type of medical treatment the child received, and even the weather at the time of the study.

After noting which individuals became ill in terms of all these factors, the two doctors looked for common denominators of high infection rates. One was age; it is no surprise to any parent that the school-age children had the highest rate of infection, most likely because they were exposed to various streptococcal strains. Whether the victims shared a room with an infected person was another factor, and the time of year was another. The majority of outbreaks were in early spring, March or April. Most other factors —weather, even the size of the family—made little difference.

Another item that affected the results was stress, both acute and chronic. About one out of four outbreaks of illness followed some sort of family crisis. The indications were that this relationship between illness and crisis was not coincidental. Meyer and Haggarty reviewed the records and checked for a stress that occurred within two weeks of an illness. Families were asked to keep diaries in which they noted particular stresses. Crises varied from a grandmother dying in one family to a family's home burning down. For example, one family was exposed to an infection at the beginning of the month by an uncle who had tonsillitis when he visited. Of the family of six, the parents and four children, only one became ill by the end of the month. She was the oldest daughter, who was under great pressure during the week of her uncle's visit to learn her catechism in time for her confirmation.

Their search showed that stress was four times as likely to precede an infection as to follow it. When throat cultures revealed a streptococcus infection, only about a fifth of the low-stress families had any disease, whereas close to half the high-stress families did. These experiments, Jemmott is careful to point out, do not prove that stress can cause an infection, only that it impairs the immune system enough to make certain individuals more susceptible. So far no one has yet deduced a treatment for the common cold on the basis of these studies. But they have helped raise researchers' consciousness of the relation of stress to illness and have prompted them to seek treatments for other infectious diseases.

Herpes

Herpes has received considerable attention in recent years. "Herpes is a particularly good model," says Robert Ader, "as it's influenced by psychosocial factors." There are two kinds of herpes. One is the type I virus that generates cold sores or fever blisters on the mouth or face. The other, more dreaded virus is the type II, which is sexually transmitted and currently extremely virulent. It is contracted by an estimated twenty-five thousand people each year. Typically the stimuli that produce an outbreak of herpes sores are exposure to sun or wind, menstruation, fever, and stress.

A characteristic of herpes is that once infected with the virus, an individual has it for life. The number of people who carry the type I virus in their system is not known, but it is suspected to be huge. Herpes has been described as the universal virus because it is so common. A puzzling and, to the psychoneuroimmunologist, significant feature of this virus is that it is unpredictable in its outbreak. After weeks, months, or even years of living in a dormant state in the body's nerves, the virus may return, erupting as sores. The factor provoking these apparently random appearances is as yet unknown, but part of the medical folklore of herpes is that the outbreaks occur in the wake of stress, such as "the woman who manifests sores only when driving a long distance to see her mother, with whom she doesn't get along," says Robert Ader.

So far only a few studies have analyzed the effect of the mind on the course of the disease. According to psychiatrist Marvin Stein of Mt. Sinai School of Medicine in New York, the studies show that herpes sores typically appear in depressed mental patients. One study of student nurses afflicted with the herpes virus discovered that those who considered themselves unhappy most of the time had more herpes outbreaks than their more cheerful classmates.

There is a double benefit of finding out the cause of herpes outbreaks. Because it has such a stress-sensitive trip wire, the virus offers tremendous potential as a tool for examining and testing theories about PNI. More significantly, because the herpes II virus is associated with cervical cancer in women victims and in birth defects in their children, finding that connection is medically important as well.

Still in its experimental stages is a program begun by psychologist Ted Grossbart, a psychologist at Beth Israel Hospital and Harvard Medical School, to use hypnotherapy to treat herpes sufferers. Diseases that affect the skin, he has found, seem to have a particularly rich history of emotional involvement. The largest organ in the body, the skin sometimes has been called the "outer rind of the ego" since its immense surface area reflects internal turmoil so graphically.

One of Grossbart's favorite illustrations of the way emotions affect the skin is a story about an airline pilot whose forehead developed herpes blisters whenever he flew over a certain canyon. Hypnotherapy brought out the fact that a friend who had substituted for him one day when he was sick crashed in that canyon. For years the pilot carried around a burden of guilt because his friend, not he, was on that flight and rode it to his death. Shortly after coming to this realization, the pilot ceased to have problems with herpes.

Another, more complex case was a man whose outbreak of genital herpes occurred each time his wife was in the fertile part of her cycle. After long discussions, Grossbart and his patient narrowed possible causes to the man's mixed feelings about becoming a parent. The pattern of herpes as punishment was a theme in his life. He felt guilty about his younger promiscuous days and thought of the herpes as his cross to bear.

For the past few years Grossbart has been concentrating his efforts on finding the emotional roots of the disease. Work in this area has gradually been coming together in a cohesive treatment strategy for a range of skin problems, from herpes to warts, the details of which we will discuss in Chapter Nine.

AIDS

An infectious disease that may someday be treatable through PNI-based therapy is Acquired Immune Deficiency Syndrome (AIDS). An extremely deadly disease with no known cure and very few options in the way of treatment, AIDS has reached epidemic proportions and continues to claim new victims, mostly gay men and drug abusers, every week. So little can be done for the AIDS sufferer that the outlook for survival is bleak.

Inspired by new psychoneuroimmunological insights a young California psychologist, Jeffrey Mandel, surveyed a group of AIDS patients in Los Angeles to determine whether relevant attitudes or behavior patterns appeared among those afflicted. Typically he found that AIDS patients "coped" by suppressing all negative emotions and practiced denial, attempting to ignore the fact that they had a deadly disease; that they had had an unusual number of occurrences of stressful events before the disease appeared; that they had felt enormous guilt about their sexual proclivities; and that they had had unresolved inner conflicts about acknowledging their homosexuality to the world.

Another finding emerged from Mandel's interviews:

It was an early impression, one that echoed some of the work that had been done elsewhere, that people who seemed to have a fighting spirit, in fact, were able to talk about their distress seemed to be doing better than those who were more stoic or passive in the wake of their diagnosis.

That raised the question to me whether or not the ability to express distress might be a mediating factor somehow in a disease which is clearly immunological, because AIDS is by definition a disease of the immune system. So that's what took it back to the psychoneuroimmunological literature. It might be an excellent illness to try to understand.

Therefore, along with others at the University of California, San Francisco School of Medicine (UCSF), Mandel is trying to devise better treatment procedures for AIDS patients and to find out which PNI insights on the value of social support, styles of coping, and specific stresses may be effective. "There's been almost no work to document how interventions may or may not make a difference in the disease progression," Mandel says.

The UCSF AIDS project is running AIDS patients through a variety of psychological tests and interviews designed to learn more about the patient's personality, life history, recent life traumas, sexual practices, and attitudes toward homosexuality. These data are cross-referenced to various immune tests on the blood, with particular attention to the ratio of helper immune cells to suppressor immune cells. The more lopsided the ratio is in favor of the suppressor cells, the more virulent the disease. Out of this research, hopes PNI pioneer Dr. George Solomon, will come a pattern of the specific PNI factors that influence AIDS and some possible directions for treatment.

That such research may offer hope for treating AIDS patients, Solomon has no doubt. As one example he mentions the cases of two gay men, both AIDS victims. One was a conservative, cultured college professor whose sex life was relatively monogamous. But he did have problems accepting his homosexuality and expressing negative emotions, such as sadness.

On one occasion he told Solomon a touching story of how, when he was a small boy, he decided to surprise his father by getting up early to go hunting with him and his friends. His father coolly walked out the door without him. "I was practically in tears as he told me this story," Solomon recalls. "And I said how did that make you feel? He said: 'I guess I must have been disappointed.' Now this is the sort of response alleged to occur in cancer-prone individuals."

By contrast, the other AIDS patient was a highly promiscuous man heavily involved in sadomasochism and bizarre sex, who frequented bars catering to like-minded individuals, drank excessively, smoked, and used more than his share of drugs. But "his self-esteem was excellent," Solomon notes. "He has a number of close friends and with a number of other sadomasochists he has formed a sadomasochist support group that meets every week to talk about their problems. He feels that his self-esteem in the past years is the highest it has ever been in his life." Interestingly, when Solomon compared the helper-suppressor T-cell ratios of the two men, the latter was in better shape. His anecdote points out the importance of the psychosocial AIDS research currently under way.

The important concluding point is that all of the research presented indicates that in most sectors of health PNI insights are potentially valuable. To be sure, surgery, antibiotics, vaccines, X rays, and painkillers play major roles in conquering or at least containing disease. But there are times when their effectiveness falls short. The search for the healer within has produced information that offers not a cure-all but a source of balm and relief. Appreciating the role the mind plays in these disease processes is the first step to developing a new body of medicine.

CHAPTER EIGHT

Cancer and the Mind

THE DOCTORS AT the Malignant Melanoma Clinic in San Francisco had noticed a disturbing pattern in many individuals stricken with melanoma, a particularly malignant form of skin cancer. They shared certain personality traits; for instance, they were model patients, compliant in the extreme. As people they were nice, excessively nice, even passive. The doctors had a hunch this pattern was not coincidental, so they asked Lydia Temoshok, a young, energetic psychologist at the University of California School of Medicine in San Francisco, to talk to the patients to attempt to detect a pattern.

Temoshok and her colleagues talked to over 150 of the clinic's patients, all melanoma sufferers. And the doctors' hunch was correct: there was a distinct group of "nice" cancer patients. They never seemed to express anger, fear, sadness, or any other negative emotions. They were the rock of stability for their families. Even in the face of cancer, they maintained this composure. "When one of them was diagnosed, they might say, 'I'm doing fine. But I'm really worried about my husband. He takes things so hard,' " explained Temoshok.

There did seem to be a distinct personality type among these patients. Because it was the exact opposite of the Type A individual, the angry, tense, hard-driving high-risk candidate for a heart attack, and different from the more relaxed, confident Type B, she dubbed this new pattern of behavior the *Type C personality*. Type Cs *always* had to feel happy and in control. The dominant characteristic of the Type C, according to Temoshok, is the nonexpression of emotion. Such a person refuses to let any negative feelings leak out. "Just as with the Type A it is not only ambition, but the hostile aspect of a person that was significant," she says, "with a Type C it is not just being nice, it's not expressing dysphoric [unpleasant] emotion."

The value of the Type C theory became apparent after interviews with the patients. Temoshok videotaped her conversations and showed them to other psychologists, who rated each individual as a Type A, B, or C. For the next year and a half Temoshok followed the course of each person's illness. The bulk of the Type Cs were concentrated in the relapsers' group, individuals whose condition became worse or who died.

After studying the nice, passive, repressed Type Cs and analyzing a small library of similar cancer-personality experiments performed over the last thirty years, Lydia Temoshok offers some tentative conclusions. One is that although no evidence indicates that personality and behavior can in any way cause cancer, the style with which a cancer patient copes can affect whether the disease continues or abates. Second, if a cancer patient has a Type C personality, "I would say that based on my research they might be at risk for having a worse outcome than might be expected on medical grounds."

On every level cancer is still a scientific mystery. It is one of the most complex and malignant diseases doctors face and is not a single ailment. Generally lumped into the category of cancer are more than one hundred diseases. Similarly, cancer has no single known cause, so that the dream of a single cure for cancer is just that, a dream.

THE DISEASE BEGINS

Cancer specialists hypothesize that at any given moment the beginning of a malignant neoplasia, a potentially deadly tumor, is stirring within the body. More often than not, it is detected and dispatched by the body's system of immune surveillance. But sometimes, for reasons still not clear, it survives and grows.

Cancer is a condition in which an abnormal body cell reproduces uncontrollably. Through a process that is not thoroughly understood, a normal body cell becomes a freak, either from a built-in genetic flaw or from a spontaneous mutation triggered by some outside force: a carcinogen, a virus, radiation, even a cosmic ray. At first the defective cells grow slowly and are highly vulnerable to attacks by the immune system. If they survive the confrontation, the newborn cancer cells become a tumor. The macrophages of the immune system may move in and engulf the enemy. If they fail, the tumor will continue to grow.

Certain chemicals and processes can interfere with the work of immune cells. For example, we now know that *corticosteroids*, biochemicals released under stress, inhibit the immune system, including the action of the macrophages. Research on coping and stress indicates that people who do not cope well in stressful situations show a decline in the activity of their natural killer cells.

Finally, Joan Borysenko has pointed out that research with animals show that mice under stress produce less *interferon*, an anticancer substance produced by T-cells. Although no one is certain why this occurs, two possible reasons are the stress-released body chemicals epinephrine and norepinephrine. When injected with these substances, animals showed impaired interferon production.

If it survives the confrontation with the immune system, the cancer does what normal tissue cannot. By a process called *angiogenesis* it stimulates the body around it to develop new blood vessels. These feed the tumor more nutrients and speed up its growth. By the time it has become a mass large enough to detect (one centimeter [a little less than half an inch] in diameter), the tumor has increased to roughly 10 billion cells. (Growth rates vary from the rapid-growing lung tumors to the slow-growing cancer of the prostate.) Left unchecked, the last stage of a cancer's evolution is to spread, or *metastasize,* invading whatever part of the body it can reach either by growing into it or by being carried there in the body's bloodstream.

Although science has not yet deciphered the precise mechanism that sets the disease in motion, some of the factors that affect susceptibility are known.

Heredity

Your genetic inheritance carries with it a built-in list of strengths and weaknesses. Epidemiologist and cancer expert Bernard Fox of the Boston University School of Medicine reports that solid evidence indicates that the disposition to lung cancer as well as to leukemia is inherited. At least five distinct types of breast cancer and at least fourteen types of colon cancers are hereditary. Less dangerous but still worrisome is skin cancer. Fair-skinned people are particularly susceptible to skin cancer, another byproduct of heredity. Further, entire races seem to have a susceptibility for or resistance to specific cancers. For example, in a region in southeast China, the residents suffer from cancer of the roof of the mouth; South African blacks have the world's highest rate of liver cancer. By contrast, breast cancer is relatively uncommon among Japanese women who live in Japan. (Japanese women in the United States, however, have approximately the same incidence of the disease as other American women, a fact that some suspect is partly due to consuming the American diet.)

Life-style

Another potent influence on susceptibility is the way people live. Unhealthy habits do their part. The most often cited self-inflicted carcinogens are tobacco and alcohol. Close to a third of all cancers have been connected to tobacco use: smoking, chewing, or sniffing. Cigarette smoke contains more than three thousand chemicals, many of them known or suspected carcinogens: arsenic, formaldehyde, vinyl chloride, and nitrites. Add drinking to that and you have taken on another 5 percent risk of head and neck cancer. High-fat and no-fiber or low-fiber diets, the food of our affluent society, have also been implicated in cancer of the uterus, ovary, breast, and colon.

Even sex habits (or lack of them) have been related to cancers. Women who have had children earlier in life tend to have lower rates of breast cancer than those who became mothers after the age of thirty-five. It has been known since the early eighteenth century that celibate women—nuns, for example—have a higher rate of breast cancer than women who have children. As if to balance that factor, cancer statistics also indicate that virgins have a lower rate of cervical cancer than women who either began having sex at a young age or have had several sex partners over the years. (Some suspect semen to be the culprit. It is known that bacteria and viruses are found in the semen; some other cancer-causing ingredients may be found there as well.)

Finally, suspected carcinogens such as the herpes I and herpes II viruses and at least five other viruses have been implicated in cancer, including the virus that causes AIDS.

Drugs

Drugs like diethylstilbestrol (DES), once given to prevent miscarriage, and immunosuppressants, used in kidney transplant patients and ironically in cancer patients, can cause cancer as well. Even Dilantin, an anticonvulsant drug commonly taken by epileptics, has been implicated in cancer of the lymph glands. By one estimate, at least ten types of drugs, from DES and certain hormones such as estrogen to amphetamines, are suspected carcinogens.

Location and Occupation

People who live in areas where the water contains high concentrations of arsenic-rich compounds, called *arsenicoles,* have a higher than average risk of skin cancer. Toxic wastes, pesticides, and other carcinogens such as dioxin that seep into local water can raise the risk of cancer in an area, as can a job working with radiation, asbestos, uranium, nickel, or cadmium. Workers in the dye industry have a high incidence of bladder cancer, and asbestos workers have a high incidence of lung cancer.

Age

Another complicating variable in measuring cancer factors is an individual's age. The odds of becoming a cancer patient increase dramatically once an individual is past the mid-sixties. One reason is that aging weakens the immune system. A more vulnerable immune system would require progressively less intense psychological factors to make it vulnerable. In effect, the significance of a life stress or psychological trauma should be different in older cancer patients than in the young.

Age can make a psychological difference as well. One German researcher, Dr. H. Becker at the University of Heidelberg's Psychosomatic Clinic, talked to forty-nine women, all of whom had received treatment for breast cancer. The patients' doctors had mentioned to Becker that the attitudes of the younger patients, those forty-eight and younger, and the older ones were distinctly different.

Following up on these suspicions, Becker found that the younger women not only had more of a violent emotional reaction to their illness, but a noticeably higher rate of life tragedies. Close to three-fourths of the younger women had experienced a tragic loss in their lives. Either a parent, sister, or brother had died, or one of the parents, usually the father, had moved out. Another common denominator was that these women had had a more difficult childhood. The parent they knew was very often cool and aloof, and more often than not, they had assumed excessive responsibility at a young age, helping to raise their younger brothers and sisters, for example.

The younger women had more psychosomatic complaints—heart trouble or stomach problems—and, unlike the older patients, an "astonishingly high" number were convinced that their cancer had psychological roots. This same group seemed to be driven and ambitious and were, at best, indifferent to marriage, motherhood, and sex; barely one of ten enjoyed sex at all.

By comparison, the older women were by all standards more normal. Their early lives were not particularly traumatic or upsetting. They enjoyed the roles of wife and mother and the experience of sex. The interesting aspect of Becker's group was that it apparently contained two groups of patients: the older women, whose cancer seemed to be a straightforward medical case of a body succumbing to a disease, and the younger women, whose emotional background suggested that more complex factors were at work.

Although this is supposed to be an age of sophistication and confidence in our technologies to "fix" almost anything, we still view cancer with a fear that is almost superstitious. Such a fear is not totally irrational; the general statistics alone are horrifying:

- Cancer affects three out of four families.

- Of all Americans living today, about 30 percent (66 million) will contract cancer in their lifetimes.

- Cancer kills more children between the ages of three and fourteen years than any other disease.

- Every day in 1983 an estimated 1,205 people, almost one person per minute, died from cancer.

We have spent billions trying to find out what cancer is. Most, if not all, of that effort has concentrated on the physical aspects of the disease. Psychological factors have been considered interesting but not relevant. The second group of women in the Becker group are the kind of cancer patients who have made psychoneuroimmunologists wonder about the nature of the relationship between the mind and cancer. The idea that the mind can influence cancer susceptibility has arrived. Now, after years of PNI research, evidence that the mind can influence the disease process is finally coalescing.

Cancer Personality

Lydia Temoshok's work is part of a body of lore on the psychology of cancer and the "cancer-prone personality." The idea that there is a cancer mind set dates to the earliest days of medicine. Psychologist Lawrence LeShan has found references going back to the eighteenth century in which the abrupt onset of cancer occurred in individuals who had recently experienced some kind of life trauma. One notable case cited by LeShan was the woman who, "upon the Death of her Daughter, underwent Great Affliction, and perceived her Breast to swell, which soon after grew Painful: at last she broke out in a most inveterate Cancer, which consumed a great Part of it in a short Time." And the second-century physician Galen noted that "melancholic" women were more prone to breast cancer than their more "sanguine" counterparts. And in 1870 the eminent British physician Sir James Paget noted: "The cases are so frequent in which deep anxiety, deferred hope and disappointment are quickly followed by the growth or increase of cancer that we can hardly doubt that mental depression is a weighty addition to the other influences that favor the development of the cancerous constitution."

In this century, scientific interest was boosted during the 1950s when psychologist Eugene Blumberg noticed the trademarks of a distinct personality among the cancer patients in a veterans' hospital in Long Beach, California: "We were impressed by the polite, apologetic, almost painful acquiescence of the patients with rapidly progressing disease as contrasted with the more expressive and sometimes bizarre personalities of those who responded brilliantly to therapy with remissions and long survival," he wrote.

Blumberg administered a psychological test to survey the cancer patients about their levels of anxiety and depression and their ability to release those pent-up emotions and tensions. When he matched his test findings with the rate at which the disease progressed, Blumberg found some interesting relationships. The patients with the fastest-growing tumors tended to be "consistently serious, over-cooperative, over-nice, over-anxious, painfully sensitive, passive, apologetic personalities" and had been all of their lives.

For example, one patient with Hodgkins disease who lived only five months had been admitted to the hospital with a heart condition. He had already admitted to the doctors that he had deliberately stopped taking his heart medicine on a few occasions, hoping that he would have a fatal heart attack. He had what Blumberg described as a willing acceptance of his cancer; it seemed to offer what he had been seeking all along: "to escape from life, its unbearable problems and stresses."

Those with slow-developing tumors, on the other hand,

seemed to have developed a way to deal with the stresses of life. That mechanism may have been part of the reason that they survived, Blumberg suggested. One woman diagnosed with breast cancer refused all conventional medical treatment, saying that it was against her religion, which gave her all the strength she needed. Ten years after her diagnosis she was still alive.

At about the time Blumberg was doing his work, New York psychologist LeShan was pursuing a similar interest in the cancer personality. He and his colleagues had interviewed 250 cancer patients and compared their life histories to other patients hospitalized for other diseases. When he analyzed the interview material, Le Shan found a striking consistency in their lives:

- Cancer patients remembered a bleak childhood, one in which they felt lonely, isolated. They had had a tense or hostile relationship with the mother, father, or both. During that part of their lives, they began to feel that any kind of deep personal relationship with anyone was not possible.

- Later, as young adults, they found something—a job, a cause, an individual—in which they made a tremendous emotional investment. That became the centerpiece of their lives.

- Then something happened to destroy it. They were fired. The beloved child left. The spouse died. In the aftershock the individual found nothing to replace that missing part of their lives and succumbed to hopeless depression. Six to eight months later, those same persons were diagnosed as having cancer.

Clues from the pasts of cancer patients also convinced psychologist Claus Bahnson, then at Jefferson Medical College in Philadelphia, that a cancer psychology was present. Of the cancer patients he interviewed, many described their parents as aloof, cold people. He found cancer patients to be emotion suppressors. They seemed to be out of touch with their own wants and needs, choosing to affect a permanent pleasant attitude and personality regardless of the bleakness of their inner lives. Part of this emotional rigidity Bahnson blamed on the strict, bloodless upbringing these people had had.

Still other researchers have tried to relate personality and attitudes to specific diseases. Scottish researcher David Kissen specialized in studying lung cancer patients and spent the better part of his scientific career trying to document personality differences between individuals who had lung cancer and those who did not. Kissen gave detailed psychological interviews to hundreds of lung cancer patients, probing into their lives, their thoughts, their feelings.

Again, when asked about childhood traumas, the cancer patients tended to gloss over events such as death of a parent, brother, or sister. Many actually had to be prodded even to recall that their mother or father had died when they were very young. Whether they failed to remember this event because they were deliberately blocking it out or because they had no deep emotional attachment to people was not clear, but one point seemed evident to Kissen: these cancer patients simply could not express their feelings. Whatever emotions they felt, they bottled up inside. A pattern began to emerge: a bleak, emotionless past and inner life seemed to be somehow involved with the onset of cancer.

If a state of mind can affect whom cancer will attack, how does it affect the outcome of a cancer already diagnosed? In other words, why do two people with the same kind of cancer, receiving identical treatment, have different outcomes? Could psychological factors make a difference? Those questions were on the minds of British psychiatrist H. Steven Greer and his colleague Dr. Tina Morris at Kings College Hospital in London. Since the early 1970s Greer and his colleagues have been following the health of breast cancer patients.

They, too, found that breast cancer patients always seemed to be holding their emotions, especially anger, in check. The patients were also the "nice" patients Temoshok described. Greer has been trying to determine which attitudes, if any, seemed to enhance the cancer's progress, and which seemed to retard it.

He has been following the patients for ten years and now thinks he has uncovered an interesting phenomenon. Those women who survived longest with no recurrence of disease were also those who initially reacted to the news they had cancer in one of two ways: denying there was anything seriously wrong with them or showing "fighting spirit," a determination to do everything possible to conquer cancer. "I can fight it and beat it" was their attitude. By contrast, women who succumbed most easily had reacted to the news of their cancer either by demonstrating a stoic, stiff-upper-lip attitude and living their lives as though nothing had changed or by having a helpless, hopeless, all-is-lost response.

Looking at a cancer patient's life history brings with it some built-in problems. One is memory. In studying the recall of life events, researchers have found that the accuracy of people's memories tends to falter for events further than six months in the past. Perfectly normal people have forgotten the deaths of friends or relatives; in fact, new events eclipse old news. The more recent past overshadows or sometimes even blocks out more distant events. For that reason, weighing the life stresses preceding the onset of cancer is difficult.

A second problem is that most studies have concentrated on people who already had cancer; and to become a cancer patient is to cease to be a "normal" person. Cancer patients may tend to reinterpret their past in light of their disease. If they think that something in their lives may have contributed to their disease, anything and everything may take on a new and weighty significance. The trauma of cancer and everything accompanying it—fear of treatment, treatment, ordeals of chemotherapy, surgery, and radiation therapy—put tremendous pressure on the human spirit as well as the body.

Finally, the disease itself may be the source of the personality and behavioral changes doctors observe. Oncologists now know from experience that one of the early symptoms of pancreatic cancer is depression; no one knows exactly why it occurs among those patients with a surprising frequency. In some instances, other cancers have spread undetected to the brains of individuals having leukemia, cancer of the lymph glands, and lung cancer. In addition, Harvard psychologist Joan Borysenko points out that cancer can affect a person's emotional state, even one's personality either by attacking the central nervous system or by skewing the delicate internal balance of hormones. Certain tumors are known to secrete hormones, some of which alter behavior or moods.

One value of these backward-looking, or *retrospective,* studies is the important questions they have raised: Are cancer patients more emotionally suppressed than other kinds of patients? Do they have more dismal childhoods? Does suffering a major personal loss make a person more cancer-prone?

The best way to find out is through a *prospective study:* recruiting

a large group of healthy people, surveying their personality characteristics, waiting twenty or thirty years to see which of them develops cancer, and then checking for common denominators present in
the beginning that might have predicted the oncoming cancer.

The advantage of this approach, of course, is that it provides
a look at patients before the disease surfaces. Through this method,
researchers avoid completely the question of whether the cancer
was the source of personality traits or whether certain events in the
patients' lives in fact preceded the cancer.

Although straightforward, this process has obvious shortcomings. The amount of money required for such a project would be
enormous, as would the number of people involved. Because only
a fraction of a group might develop cancer over a limited period of
time, the initial group collected for such a study would have to be
large. How large? When he was working at the National Cancer
Institute, cancer expert and behavioral epidemiologist Bernard Fox
calculated that a dedicated researcher would have to follow ten
thousand people for at least twenty years. This raises the second
problem: the logistics of following ten thousand people for two
decades would not be simple, especially given that the average
American moves every seven years.

A workable alternative has been to use information from long-
term studies already underway. Probably the best known was
begun at The Johns Hopkins University Medical School in 1946
under the direction of Dr. Caroline Thomas (now an emeritus professor of medicine). The thesis of her study was simple: that just as
certain physical clues, such as high blood pressure and serum cho-
lesterol levels, indicate whether a person is at high risk for heart
disease, psychological characteristics—personality traits, behaviors,
family attitudes—may be markers of future troubles.

With that goal, Thomas selected a sample of Johns Hopkins
medical students who were graduates between 1948 and 1964, more
than thirteen hundred people in all. She administered a battery of
physical and psychological tests and took elaborate family histories
from each. In the years that followed their graduation, the doctors
kept Dr. Thomas updated on their medical histories by mail.

Although Thomas's original intent was to concentrate on coronary heart disease, she later included cancer for comparison, assuming it to be the least likely disease to be affected by behavior.
Finally, in the mid-1970s Thomas sorted through the data she had

been patiently collecting for the preceding thirty plus years.

By 1978 two hundred of the graduates had serious illnesses: hypertension, coronary heart disease, and cancer (forty-eight cancer patients in all). As she searched her records of these men's student days, curiously regular findings emerged from the files of the cancer patients, as well as those of individuals who became mentally ill or who committed suicide. These students had scored noticeably low on psychological tests that concerned their family relationships. Particularly low was their score on the closeness-to-parents scale.

Typically the cancer patients described themselves as emotionally detached from their parents and mentioned that their parents themselves had been disagreeable to one another. In general, more negative attitudes about the family prevailed among the cancer patients than among any other group in the study.

The pattern has continued to hold. Many of the men now in their forties and fifties who, while in their twenties, described a rather bleak family life on Thomas's questionnaire now have cancer. Her findings, she says, echo the conclusions drawn by other studies: Claus Bahnson's work, which postulated a sense of alienation among cancer patients whose source is the individual's childhood; and LeShan's description of cancer patients as people who habitually bottle up their emotions, particularly their negative ones. These characterizations meshed neatly with those of some of Thomas's doctors: a pattern formed early in the life of the subjects that physiologically somehow enhanced their risk of cancer. Emotionally this trait manifested itself as depression.

Depression

Is it possible that depression may have a carcinogenic effect? Many of those individuals doing PNI research in cancer believe that it can. Some of the evidence for such a thesis is derived from *pseudoprospective studies:* research following the case histories of people who have symptoms suggestive of cancer. Such symptoms would include a lump in the breast, a spot on the lung, an abnormal Papanicolaou's test (Pap smear).

Before a final diagnosis is made and the presence of cancer has been confirmed, the researchers talk to the patients and gather as much information as possible about their personality and psychological history to attempt to predict which individuals will develop cancer. The rationale for this approach is that if our states of mind can influence the body's susceptibility, then attempting to determine whether high-risk individuals can be predicted through psychological indicators would be useful.

One of the most impressive efforts of this kind was made by Doctors Arthur Schmale and Howard Iker at the University of Rochester. Schmale and Iker had noticed that cancer and other diseases appeared after individuals experienced certain high-stress situations, for example, death of the spouse, and that the individuals simply seemed to cave in to the stress. For their subjects they chose a group of women whose Pap tests (the standard tests for cervical cancer) revealed what were described as "suspicious" cells. They were asked to return to the hospital for more tests. The researchers hoped to predict from their psychological assessment which of the women would turn out to have cancer before the diagnosis was made. Their prediction was that the women who would be diagnosed with cancer would report having responded to some major life upheaval with hopelessness.

Schmale and Iker gave a battery of psychological tests to fifty-one women in all. After the tests the doctors asked each to talk about herself for about an hour. They were looking for the expression of depression and hopelessness, defined by Schmale as "a feeling of frustration, despair or futility perceived as coming from a loss of satisfaction for which the individual himself assumed complete and final responsibility by a sense of frustration that one has failed miserably at accomplishing anything in life. . . ."

On the basis of these tests and interviews, Schmale and Iker predicted that eighteen women would develop cancer and that thirty-three would not. Their forecasts proved remarkably accurate: of those eighteen marked as cancer patients, eleven had the disease. Of the thirty-three others, twenty-five were cancer-free. Their findings were based solely on the degree of hopelessness a woman showed in the face of stress, not the amount of stress each woman had survived.

One woman was tolerating an unfaithful husband "because of the children," another "because he needs me." By comparison, when one of the cancer-free patients found herself in a similar situation with her boyfriend, she ended the relationship. These were all conditions or events that existed during the six months prior to the diagnosis.

Although years have passed since his formal study, Schmale continues to work with cancer patients and still sees some of these same traits today. He reports that many, not all, cancer patients have a willingness to please, an overeagerness to comply that is typical and offers a little insight into the reason they chose to remain in a helpless situation. "They're very devoted. They want to help. You see it over and over again," says Schmale, "the cancer patient being the 'good' patient. I think that's part of the cancer patient's personality." Those he had marked as high-risk patients tended to be overly conscientious and self-sacrificing. They were also more depressed than the noncancerous patients.

Depression has also emerged as a recurrent theme in research into the psychological factors surrounding cancer, first from copious 1957–58 test data analyzed by two University of Chicago researchers, Linas Bieliauskas and Richard Shekelle; they recently reported the results of the psychological tests given seventeen years earlier to over two thousand workers at a Chicago Western Electric plant. The two men were focusing on the dominant moods and attitudes of each worker indicated by the tests.[1]

With the results in hand, Bieliauskas and Shekelle tracked down information about the current health of the participants. Sixty had died from cancer. Bieliauskas and Shekelle tried to determine which common variables characterized the cancer patients, whether they smoked or drank, for example. The noticeable characteristic they all tended to share was depression, not sufficient to require hospitalization or medical attention, but greater than that of the average person. Reducing the data to statistics, Shekelle concludes that those who died of cancer were twice as likely to have had high depression scores on their tests as those who had no cancer at all. Furthermore, the higher cancer rates among the "depressed" group could not be explained on the basis of their drinking or smoking habits.

THE MIND SET MIRAGE

Given all this evidence, one is tempted to postulate a cancer mind set. These data seem to present a psychological profile of some cancer patients. Among the most common stresses and psychological traits associated with cancer are the following:

- experiencing loss of an important relationship or a significant person, thing, or position in life

- being a rigid, conforming person with an overly critical attitude toward oneself

- having a disturbed or emotionally sterile relationship with one's parents

- lacking satisfactory emotional outlets—a habit of bottling up or suppressing anger and other strong emotions

- having a poor ability to deal with stressful life change, a sense of hopelessness or helplessness in the face of stress

- being depressed, not necessarily so severe as to require professional help, but sufficient to register far above average on a psychological test.

Although some of the clues to mental influences over cancer are impressive, more research is needed. It is easy to be seduced by study results, points out Dr. Bernard Fox, an epidemiologist at Boston University Medical Center and expert on such studies. When he was at the National Cancer Institute, Fox reviewed studies linking psychological states to cancer on the basis of their being good, bad, or indifferent examples of scientific research.[2]

After digesting the contents of a few decades' work on the subject, Fox pointed out that it is difficult to find an emotion that is not related to cancer by one study or another, sometimes by the most slender thread of proof. Only one state of mind, depression, seemed to recur with some frequency, but nevertheless Fox is cautious about generalizing. In most of the studies, depression did not predict the development of cancer; it just occurred more frequently than other traits in cases of the disease.

Some of the evidence from the studies he finds unconvincing, for example, the study by Caroline Thomas. First, it was originally designed to indicate susceptibility to heart disease. Cancer appeared by chance. Second, the number of cancer cases has been too small, only about fifty, too few to be highly significant yet. Finally, she studied so many variables in her research that by chance alone a researcher would find relationships between them that appeared significant.

Aside from the flaws of some of the research, Fox and others suggest that basic questions have yet to be answered: Does stress or a cancer personality cause the disease? If an attitude or mind set influences the disease, how does it do it?

In theory, stress could directly cause cancer by setting off changes in the neuroendocrine system, causing a biochemical reaction that could transform normal cells into malignant ones.

Alternatively, stress could weaken the immune system sufficiently that it could not hold a forming tumor in check, allowing a small, controllable cancer to become a large, fast-growing one.

A third possibility is that stress speeds up the rate of growth of an established cancer. The tumor starts to grow quickly, either through a direct influence on the tumor or through impairment of the antitumor elements in the immune system.

That a specific life event or series of traumatic life events is responsible for the tumor, according to Bernard Fox, does not make sense. Some life stress studies looked no further back in a person's past than six months to a year and a half for significant events. Although almost everyone knows someone who developed cancer after a major life stress, the death of a spouse, the cancer was probably already present. A cancer cell takes years to multiply and grow into a detectable tumor. For lung cancer the latency period can run from two years, in fast-growing cancers, to five years. For breast tumors the latency is at least five years and as long as eleven.

In addition, other possible explanations account for the change in moods and attitudes that sometimes accompany the disease. According to cancer expert Daphne Panagis of the West Coast Cancer Foundation in San Francisco, certain psychological characteristics that occur with cancer may be coincidental; or may indicate reverse causality, the cancer influencing the mood change. In other words, some common cause may have contributed to the tumor growth and caused the personality traits to appear.

Take a child in a family with a high mortality rate from cancer.

Suppose one of his parents dies from the disease at a relatively early age. That child could grow up ignored by the surviving parent, who is grieving over his or her dead spouse. Deprived of the attention of the grief-stricken parent, the child might develop into a maladjusted, depressed adult. Should he develop cancer later in life one could say that the family history of having the disease was a potent factor both in his developing cancer and in the shaping of his personality.

THE SECRET OF CANCER SURVIVORS

The fact remains that people do survive savage bouts with cancer, sometimes against all medical odds. This circumstance raises the question of the capacities they have or actions they take that distinguish them from other cancer patients.

At the University of Pittsburgh, psychologist Sandra Levy has been trying to find out. Over the past few years she has been trying to see if there was any truth to the medical folklore that the nicer the patient, the shorter the lifespan. Are experts such as Schmale and Iker correct that the nice, passive patients do not do so well as those who are more aggressive?

Working with immunologist Ronald Herberman and breast cancer expert Marc Lippman of the National Cancer Institute, Levy studied seventy-five breast cancer patients, noting their progress for a year, paying particular attention to their attitudes and health. She chose a group of women with recurrent breast cancer, patients not expected to live long. By the year's end, six of the women had died.

Those who tended to be cancer survivors, that is, whose condition was stable, also complained the most. Levy and Herberman examined blood from the outspoken patients and found that women who complained about more psychiatric problems, depression or anxiety, also had more active anticancer natural killer cells. They also had better prognoses, suggesting that attitude helped mobilize the anticancer elements of their immune system.

Curiously, Dr. Locke's research on the same kind of cells gave a seemingly opposite result. Dr. Locke and his colleagues found that among a group of healthy college students those who complained most about depression and anxiety, who had the same kinds of negative feelings as those of Dr. Levy's patients, had less active natural killer cells.

Is this result contradictory? Is one of the studies woefully inaccurate? Not necessarily, according to Chicago psychologist Linas Bieliauskas. In struggling to understand the meaning of these apparent contradictions, Dr. Bieliauskas offered an explanation. It is abnormal for perfectly healthy students to complain of anxiety and depression; however, it is abnormal for cancer patients not to complain. Normal, adaptive behavior for healthy people is different from that of sick people. For someone who is ill, complaining is reasonable; the sick role sanctions it. After all, the patient certainly has valid cause to complain.

Fortunately, some well-designed efforts to incorporate psychoneuroimmunological insights into treatments that are experimental but promising are under way. At University of California, San Francisco, psychologist Lydia Temoshok has already adapted some of the insights in her work with Type C cancer patients, individuals who avoid expressing emotions, especially negative emotions. She stresses that her approach is only experimental and still evolving. Nevertheless, she has been getting encouraging results.

Part of Temoshok's approach has been to try to enhance the cancer patients' body awareness—to put them in touch with the realities of the disease—and to effect positive changes in their behavior. One case she remembers particularly was a "nice" Type C man, a leukemia patient, who was told that he was most likely to live only a few more months. "The thing we worked on strongly was to have him recognize what his needs are, including his bodily needs." He simply chose to ignore basic needs for resting or for taking care of himself. "He wouldn't even know when he was tired," Temoshok offers as one example. "One night he stayed up for hours sorting out his medical bills and collapsed into bed exhausted from the strain of pushing himself."

He exhibited the Type C nice-guy style of behavior that Temoshok hoped to change. "There was an example almost every minute," Temoshok recalls with some amused exasperation:

He'd be talking with me and a nurse would come into the hospital room and say, "Could I give you a shot now?" And he would say: "Oh, fine, sure." And I would say *what?* And he would catch himself and would say "Umm, what I mean to say is we're talking now; could you come back later?"

Or we'd be making an appointment, and I'd say, "What time would you like me to come back?" And he'd say "What time is convenient for you?" And I would come back with: "No. What time would *you* like me to come back? I have this hour"—I would give him a time—"free." He would hesitate. And I'd say, "Now there is something wrong with that hour, isn't there? Why don't you tell me what it is?" He'd reply: "I was planning to see someone else then." I would say, "Why didn't you say that?"

It was a painful process of redirecting almost everything he was doing with his life. For the first time in his life he was taking the time to think about his own physical and emotional needs. He learned to use the cancer as an excuse to express his own wants. He might say: "I'm really feeling tired now because of the treatments. Could you come back tomorrow?" That is a mild-mannered statement but he would never say that before.

Changing a characteristic as evanescent as an attitude made quantifying whether the therapy made a difference in the course of his illness difficult, but indications suggest that it made at least a positive difference to him. Faced with a serious disease, he finally asked to talk to the son from whom he had been aloof.

Coincident with his therapy, his health began to improve. Before the program, his blood platelet count, one indicator of the strength of his immune system, was dropping almost daily and the prognosis was poor. As Temoshok worked with the man, his leukemia reversed. His immune system seemed to rally and to reassert control. "He got better and better and better," she recalls with some satisfaction. "His blood counts improved every day. Now he has left the hospital. He still has problems, but he's doing okay."

She makes no claims to have cured him or effected a miracle, only to have improved his ability to cope.

Temoshok has also used biofeedback, not to train her patients to change their bodies so much as show them how it registers their emotions. She attached one woman from Utah with malignant melanoma to a biofeedback machine and asked her to talk about the last time she was angry. "That's an important question with these people," Temoshok explains. As the woman talked, her voice showed no expression and she might even say that the anger-provoking incident really didn't bother her. But biofeedback readings belied her statements; the machine registered her tension.

The biofeedback offered a valuable object lesson: "It allowed her to feel that this was another important reason for expressing anger—because *not* doing so was dangerous to her," Temoshok says. "But she had to see it demonstrated before it was justified."

Temoshok concedes that her work is still in the groping early stages of any experimental effort. She suggests that attempting to help cancer patients deal with the disease on any level, even psychological, when the procedure is characterized by intelligence and sensitivity, can effect a positive change.

Writing on "The Influence of Mind on Cancer," Dr. Alastair Cunningham, an oncologist at the Ontario Cancer Institute in Canada, has noted that no scientific evidence indicates that a psychotherapeutic approach to treating cancer affects the outcome. However, the evidence that exists, he says, warrants trying them, with so much to gain and so little to lose.

Is the cure for cancer, which has eluded the best efforts of science, in the mind? Do individuals have carcinogenic personalities, reactions, and moods? In spite of claims to the contrary, no one has truly broken the code of the mind-cancer link. So complicated a relationship is elusive. Even so, we can comfortably make some broad statements about it:

- No scientific evidence indicates that stress, emotions, or personality style can *cause* cancer.

- However, after decades of relegation to the fringes of medicine, the idea that attitudes and mental states may affect the course of cancer is gaining acceptance. The strongest, although not yet convincing, evidence suggests that depression in particular may be a risk factor. Less definitive but still intriguing evidence suggests that disturbed family relationships may contribute to susceptibility. Finally, it is possible that emotions pave the way for the onset of cancer by suppressing the potency of the immune system.

- It is not yet possible to predict which individuals will develop cancer or even the way cancer patients will be able to fight it solely by probing an individual's psyche for clues: too many psychological and behavioral undercurrents of the disease must first be sorted out.

When moving into the shadow land between the mind and the body in regard to so complex a disease as cancer, it is easy to feel overwhelmed. However, enough is now known about the mechanisms of the body and mind to justify trying, as Lydia Temoshok has, to use the findings that PNI research has generated. Unfortunately, rushing psychoneuroimmunology into the mainstream of medicine has pitfalls. As Chapter Nine indicates, problems arise when many people in their enthusiasm too quickly embrace what are touted as the principles of PNI in the unrelated and sometimes dangerous therapeutic practice known as holistic medicine.

CHAPTER NINE

Finding the Healer Within

The setting is *Star Trek* with a little Disney. You sit in a high-tech easy chair as a group of computer-animated images drift by on a large projection screen. Representations of white blood cells flash before your eyes to help you visualize your immune system fighting off the cancer. The walls are studded with soundproofing bumps to minimize distractions from outside the room. A mixture of bland music and surf sounds—"white noise"—is piped into your ears through a special headset. Embedded somewhere in the noise are healthful subliminal messages targeted to reach your "decision-making right brain," a multicolored brochure informs anyone who writes for information.

You will spend a part of each day of your twenty-one-day stay in this room, watching the cartoon images, listening to the sounds. The rest of the time you will be learning to overcome the fear of cancer, learning some basic facts about nutrition and exercise, attending therapy sessions.

The routine is standard in this unusual, but not unique center, dedicated solely to teaching people afflicted with cancer to rehabilitate their immune system to "detect cancerous cells and effectively kill and remove them." No chemotherapy, no radiation therapy here: the medicine is your mind. Its power comes from concentrating on the animated figures on the screen. You are not only the patient but the doctor. Throughout this health spa regimen you will be fighting for your life.

The director of the center talks glibly yet vaguely of unnamed Nobel Laureates involved in the techniques used ("there are even scientists who have won Nobel prizes for some of the discoveries contained in the animation"). He makes general references to some current medical research and, while promising no sure cure, hints at many successes. (Unnamed studies of similar techniques, he says, show that his techniques can double "the life expectancy of colon, lung, and breast cancer [patients]. . . .") The cost of this twenty-one day stay is $1,900. The director plans to open a chain of such treatment centers offering this dramatic holistic therapy.

By contrast, in the late 1980s a group of therapists at the Washington School of Psychiatry, themselves cancer victims, decided to try their own imagery experiment with cancer patients. The group was started by the director of the school, the late Dr. Robert Kvarnes, who taught the group to use guided imagery in an attempt to try to influence their immune system.

In a typical imagery session, Kvarnes suggested the group visualize a descent, down a tunnel or long, winding staircase, until they found a thread. That thread led through a maze of rooms to a dark inner chamber, one with a "cancer presence." In the mythology of the imagery session each person had a crystal to ward off any evils, and a wizard on demand would help the image maker handle any crises that arose. Once inside that innermost chamber and face to face with the cancer, each person was free to plan an individual strategy of attack.

For one cancer patient, that search led to increasingly smaller rooms and finally to a small cavelike chamber, where the search by the light of the crystal illuminated a small worm, the cancer, which burned with a mysterious fire. Somehow he had to squelch that fire. The goal of the program was simple: to determine whether these exercises could in any way influence the course of the disease. The patients were all volunteers, the program was strictly experimental, and no fees were charged.

For technical assistance, Kvarnes enlisted help from immunological experts, among them Nicholas Hall, a neuroendocrinologist at the Department of Biochemistry at George Washington University. Hall explained to the small group the basics of the way the immune system works. The group constituted a cross section of cancer cases—ovarian cancer, cancer of the prostate, lung cancer—and numbered only about ten people. (In the end, only three people continued doing daily imagery experiments and keeping a diary of their simultaneous thoughts and feelings.) Hall and his colleagues also took blood samples from each person, studying the virulence with which their immune systems resisted cancer cells, and looked for traces of other biochemicals, such as thymosin, the secretion of the thymus gland that plays an important role in immunology.

As an experiment, it had some unusual problems. Hall found maintaining his role as scientist-observer difficult. Blood samples were taken and measured for immune potency. At the end of the first six months, the people were told for the first time whether they were performing well or poorly on the immune-imagery scale. Revealing the initial results changed the experiment: "We got some spectacular results and the individuals who had given up on it, thinking they were wasting their time, now had an incentive to pick it up again," says Hall, a cheery, effervescent man. "At that point we were beginning to become a part of the study itself." Today he characterizes the procedure only as "interesting." He offers no suggestions of cancer cures in his conversation.

The two groups, Kvarnes's and the cancer therapy entrepreneur's, provide an interesting study in contrast. Both seek to use the same inner resources to combat the similar diseases in very similar ways. The techniques are theatrical. Even the motivation of the two groups, to a certain degree, is similar: the therapy franchiser is unshakably convinced he has formularized the healer within and can make it available to anyone. By contrast, Hall and his colleagues make no claims except that they have had a glimmering of some healing potential and hope to study and understand the process. Although Hall remains fascinated by the study results, he has no illusion that the specific images worked any biochemical magic. If anything made a difference, he says, it was that the cancer patients were doing something, like the rats that had control, to alleviate their medical situation. "I would suspect for some, religion might play the same kind of role. Still others might accomplish the same thing with biofeedback or exercise."

These two groups represent two extremes of much of medicine today. More and more, doctors and patients are looking beyond traditional medicine to alternative therapies and, in some instances, are getting encouraging results. The emphasis in psychoneuroimmunology on searching beyond the traditional therapies and concepts of the medical school classroom has made the art and science of healing more complex, more challenging, more potentially rewarding, and for the time being a little chaotic.

At one time scientific medicine had monolithic control over the art and science of healing. John Burnham, professor of history at Ohio State University, has described the status of medicine in an essay, "American Medicine's Golden Age: What Happened to It?" At one time physicians had a sacerdotal role, according to Burnham. People expected much more of them than of other professionals. And much of the doctor's prestige came from the aura bestowed on them by "priestly functioning as they went through medical ceremonies and acted as wise and trusted personages." This mythic image of the doctor was kept alive by pop culture icons such as *Marcus Welby*, the wise, fatherly physician-healer able to listen and heal. But even as Marcus Welby was being beamed into peoples' living rooms, medicine was experiencing a fall from grace. The public's confidence in the profession began to fade in the late 1950s and early 1960s. During those years voices of criticism were directed at many of America's revered totems: the city, the large family, the automobile, any and all traditional institutions.

Some of the criticism of medicine was caused by changes in the perceived effectiveness of medical technology. The omnipotent stature of medicine and its practitioners was crumbling. Although the magic bullets had practically eliminated diseases such as tuberculosis and polio, doctors seemed powerless to stop chronic killers such as heart disease and cancer, the two most common causes of death. New strains of bacteria, maddeningly resistant to the antibiotic wonder drugs, appeared. Added to these factors, the postwar surge of psychosomatic medicine made a powerful case for an important force in disease being the mind. This trend revealed something out of reach of the technology of medical science: psychosomatic illness.

Worse still was the realization that medicines and prescriptions were not inevitably benign and helpful: Doctors did not always know best. Pregnant women prescribed supposedly harmless tranquillizers were giving birth to gravely deformed children in the United States and England. A series of sudden deaths of small children was traced to a commonly prescribed antibiotic, chloramphenicol. Bad news continued through the 1960s: the carcinogenic effects of DES, the perceived overprescription of tonsillectomies and Cesarean sections, and the opposition of the American Medical Association (AMA) to Medicare. The image of doctors as moral and social superiors in society was tarnished by conspiracies of silence among M.D.s, their wealth, and their materialism. The image of the doctor as shaman and healer gave way to the doctor as corporation: John Doe, M.D., Inc.

And there was also the financial factor. During the 1960s the American public began losing its patience with the way in which health care was dispensed: it was getting too expensive. Between 1950 and 1965, the cost of medical care in the United States quadrupled, from $10 billion to $40 billion, and in relative figures rose from 4 to 6 percent of the gross national product (GNP). By 1970, the cost had risen to $70 billion, more than 7 percent of the GNP. By 1983 Americans were spending 10.5 percent of the GNP on medical care.

The rules of reimbursement for health care also encouraged greater impersonality in some aspects of medicine. Health insurance plans typically paid doctors more if the same service were performed in a hospital than in an office. Since certain procedures were more "cost-productive," they were logically favored. "As a result, some services, like cataract surgery, are financial 'winners' because they pay more than they cost to produce," says Harvard sociologist Paul Starr, "while other services, like talking to a patient are 'losers' because they pay less than what they cost."

Another powerful and sometimes overlooked factor in demythologizing the doctor as the omniscient healer was the evolution of a more sophisticated patient. People had now become consumers. Once rare, malpractice suits began to become more and more common. Loyalties to individual doctors faded. Patients began to shop around for their physicians. Ironically, says Burnham, this situation

most favored the technically oriented specialist, usually not re-
nowned for bedside manner, and least favored the family practitioner.

One of the chief reasons patients became more outspoken
about the quality and nature of health care was the women's movement of the 1960s. Infuriated by the sometimes cavalier way they
had been treated by male doctors, more and more women became
extremely well-informed patients. They learned to perform gynecological self-examinations, set up underground abortion referral
services, and encouraged women to demand drug-free Lamaze
childbirth techniques, or childbirth at home under the supervision
of a doctor or even a lay midwife.

Gynecological exams, childbirth, and abortion became political
issues. The self-help text *Our Bodies, Ourselves*, published by the
Boston's Women's Health Collective, became the movement's man-
ifesto. That sociopolitical force spearheaded the trend among
women patients to assume more active roles in their health care.

Another part of the cultural fallout of the sixties was the concern over what could be called "superhealth," a positive state of
being. Better than merely feeling all right, it was a higher state of
fitness: special diets, special exercises, a new fascination with East-
ern religions and rituals with their mind- and body-control techniques encouraged experimentation and, in general, a view of health
as being more than disease-free. Although it was possible to achieve
a higher level of health, the process required a more eclectic approach to healing. The glory days of the magic bullet were gone.
Becoming and staying well presented a complex challenge that required going outside traditional Western medicine.

This spirit of therapeutic dissent, as Paul Starr calls it, encouraged the birth of a medical counterculture with an interesting mix
of political views, from the liberal feminists and the consumerist
movements that sought to give patients the right to choose their
own treatment, to more conservative right-wing groups who took
a particular interest in legalizing freedom of choice to have the
controversial cancer treatment, laetrile.

The rebellious attitude against conventional medicine is not
new, Starr points out, but a throwback to an attitude that prevailed
in the last century. "Just as nineteenth-century critics called for a
democratization of medical knowledge ('every man his own doctor'), so did the new advocates of health care."

This attitude was neatly complemented by what Burnham calls the "resurgence of romantic individualism." Looking beyond standard technologies, ancient therapies were rediscovered in the 1960s. The ancient Chinese art of acupuncture was brought to the United States after *New York Times* reporter James Reston's stories about his operation, as were the self-pacifying benefits of Transcendental Meditation, which was imported from India.

These nontraditional therapies gained new legitimacy after a few courageous researchers used the conventional techniques of Western science to study similar phenomena. Psychologist Neal Miller at the Rockefeller University in New York taught biofeedback to animals; research at the Menninger Clinic in Topeka, Kansas, pioneered scientifically refined biofeedback techniques; at Harvard Medical School, cardiologist Dr. Herbert Benson developed his TM-like method for evoking the relaxation response.

The net result was that by the late 1970s and early 1980s physicians had lost much of their high status. As one sign of that change, a Harris Poll conducted in 1966 showed that 73 percent of those who responded had a great deal of confidence in physicians; by 1982 that confident majority had shrunk to only 32 percent. Traditional medicine had lost its monopoly on the craft of healing. Both patients and practitioners became more receptive to alternative therapies: A new philosophy of medicine began to take shape out of the reevaluation and dissent. It was the antithesis of Descartes's mind-body dualism and was based on the idea that each patient is a unique individual made up of body, mind, and spirit and should be diagnosed and treated according to the way these elements interact with each other and with the patient's environment.

Such ideas have already had real impact on the subtler aspects of medical practice: causing doctors to view the patient as a person, not as a medical case; making physicians aware that they can affect patients' health in the way they interact with them; showing doctors that they can help patients achieve health by teaching them to remain healthy and encouraging them to collaborate with their doctors, rather than to receive treatments passively.

Medical schools are reflecting this new awareness. At Brown University, for example, a newly initiated course is designed to help medical students learn to interact with patients. Students talk to actors playing the role of patients in videotaped sessions and then review the videotape to learn whether they communicated well or poorly.

Since 1979 two faculty members of the Mt. Sinai School of Medicine, Doctors Richard Gorlin and Howard Zucker, have been teaching a course in humanistic medicine. The course attempts to make interns and medical students aware of their own feelings about patients and the way those feelings affect the kind of care the patients receive. Very often a doctor whose patient has a terminal illness or a chronic, incurable disease feels impotent or frustrated. As a result the physician may avoid discussing the illness with the patient or may avoid the patient altogether. "It is critical to realize that even when there is no further specific therapy available, there are constructive things that can and should be done to help the patient and the family endure the experience," Gorlin and Zucker noted in *The New England Journal of Medicine.* Both report that since the program has been initiated, the atmosphere of Mt. Sinai Medical Center has noticeably improved, largely, suggest the authors, because the young doctors have "gained the strength to feel [their] humanity and to deal with it."

Some of the credit for this new awareness belongs to the ideals of holistic medicine, that each patient is a unique entity of body and spirit, and both elements need nurturing and attention. The concept of holism is traditionally traced back to a 1926 book, *Holism and Evolution,* by a South African philosopher, Jan Smuts. His work set the tone for the holistic movement by challenging, for good reason, conventional science and medicine's reductionist trait of oversimplifying complex systems and organisms.

Although the holistic ideal has effected some improvements in the philosophy of medicine, its contributions to the science of medicine have been erratic. "That's the problem," points out University of Rochester's Dr. Robert Ader. "There is a legitimate *concept* of holistic medicine, and then there is the holistic medicine *movement,* which I view essentially as anti-intellectual, anti-scientific."

As a science it offers a vague, unfocused approach to healing. As Dr. Andrew Weil, a Harvard-educated observer and sometime practitioner of alternative medicines, has said: "There's a lot of inconsistency in the holistic health movement. It ranges from ideas and ideals that I think are solid to very unscientific acceptance of procedures just because they're unorthodox."

The basic problem physicians have had is applying this philosophy. In trying to treat the *holos,* many holistic practitioners have committed the same sins they have attributed to conventional medicine. A chief difficulty of the holistic movement is its exclusionary attitude toward the realm of scientific medicine and its uncritical, anti-intellectual, antimedical, and antiscientific stance.

Enthusiasts support the idea with a fervor unmatched in conventional medicine. For example, in *The New England Journal of Medicine,* Dr. Faith Fitzgerald of the University of California, Davis, Medical Center, discussed her observations on holistic apostles and their various therapies when she traveled the talk-show circuit. Most of those she saw and met were "true believers," sincere, well-meaning individuals who were convinced they had *the answer* and spoke with the fervor of the converted. Unfortunately the answer varied from one proselytizer to the next.

For these believers, Fitzgerald noticed, illness takes on metaphysical proportions. People become ill "because they didn't eat right or exercise enough, or they had negative thoughts. Sin for them is 'un-Natural' action and sickness, the wrath of that offended deity." In short, Fitzgerald emerged from the experience convinced that for many, holistic medicine "is a religion. And as such stands on a different plane of thought than does science." Practicing holistic medicine is more a matter of belief than of scientific conviction.

Citing one example, Fitzgerald says that one vitamin therapy proponent challenged her with: "It's not enough for you doctors to say, 'There's no evidence that this works. You have to test it, to prove scientifically that it doesn't work.'" That attitude distinguishes the holistic movement from the holistic idea: little or no patience for scientific proof. Many believers see the scientific method only as a weapon of destruction wielded by suspicious and hostile doctors, eager to protect their turf at all costs.

When asked why only limited testing precedes the use of therapies or cures, people working in holistic health often say that researching why one or another therapy is effective is not their responsibility. As a result, some holistic healers offer treatments that are not only unconventional but unproven.

Another question about offering unproven treatments is whether holistic practitioners have a right to charge fees for such therapies. Even if the therapies are harmless, the ethical question lingers. When individuals consult conventional doctors, they expect that once a diagnosis is made, there is a reasonable probability that treatment will be successful, largely because the treatment has been tried with a better than average rate of success. (Furthermore, when patients are treated at university hospitals with experimental treatments, they generally are not charged for the unproven treatment.) In matters of life and health, hunches that a certain therapy is "good" may not be enough.

Another danger is total belief in the harmlessness of holism. Any treatment involves risks as well as benefits. For its flaws, allopathic (that is, traditional) medicine minimizes risks as much as possible. (A basic ancient tenet of allopathic medicine is *Primum non nocere*, first do no harm.) Unfortunately holists often choose to ignore the potential dangers associated with their methods. Probably the best way to exemplify the pitfalls of this approach to medicine is to investigate holistic therapies for cancer.

THE HOLISTIC TOUCH

Dozens of different kinds of alternative cancer treatments are available today. It is instructive to examine treatments themselves and the people who seek them out. University of Pennsylvania psychologist Barrie Cassileth and her associates talked to more than three hundred cancer patients to find out why they chose to go to alternative cancer centers. Although none of the centers claimed to offer cancer cures, the largest percentage of those who went to them nevertheless expected a cure or remission. Most of the people were drawn to these alternative treatments because they seemed nontoxic, especially when compared to chemotherapy, radiology, and surgery.

Two interesting sidelights emerged from the survey. One was that there were few charlatans among those giving treatments; most were sincere. The second was that the patients who sought out these treatments were not the uninformed, desperate, naïve cancer patients they are often assumed to be. Most were described as being well educated and continuing to use conventional therapy along with their unorthodox treatments.

For a closer look at the treatments themselves, Michael Lerner, a clinical psychologist, spent three years visiting more than thirty "complementary cancer centers" all over the world. The therapies they offered varied from programs that used special herbs and macrobiotics to programs like the one mentioned earlier that used cancer-fighting mental images. Lerner found that the therapies had no discernible effect on ten percent of the patients, but that about 40 percent thought they experienced some sort of temporary improvements in the quality of their lives. About the same percentage said they felt slightly more lasting specific medical benefits, for example, a period of weeks, months, or even years in which they lived disease-free. Finally a small minority, about ten percent of the people surveyed had a partial or complete remission of cancer.

On reviewing his three-year scientific pilgrimage, Lerner offered some personal conclusions. Some of the therapies seem to help the patients physically, psychologically, or both; yet nowhere did he find anything approaching a cure for cancer. Practically no scientific evidence indicated that any of these programs effected the cures they sometimes claimed.

A good example of one of the better-known holistic centers is the Simonton Cancer Center of radiotherapist O. Carl Simonton. We single it out for several reasons: it is carefully managed and reputable. Simonton himself has good credentials: he is a licensed M.D. and a Board-certified radiotherapist with several years of experience treating cancer patients with conventional radiotherapy. From a holistic perspective, the Simonton program has been widely praised.

Located in Pacific Palisades, California, the Center describes itself as a study and treatment center for the emotional aspects of cancer. To receive the therapy, cancer patients travel to California and there, for $2,700 (covered by most medical plans as a psychotherapy cost), each visitor, accompanied by a supportive companion, undergoes a five-day group program that combines traditional and nontraditional techniques. It is all designed to affect the course of the disease, the quality of life of the cancer patients, and ultimately the quality of the patient's death.

Over the five days people learn techniques to help them manage the disease: meditation and a special kind of imagery technique Simonton and his former wife, Stephanie Matthews-Simonton, pioneered. Patients attend lectures on stress, nutrition, hope, hopelessness, dealing with the recurrence of the disease, and facing the prospect of death. Simonton's goal is to teach attitudes and skills that may improve the cancer patient's quality of life over the next two years. To illustrate to the patients the kinds of untapped powers they have at their disposal, he and his staff do a firewalk, across a bed of live coals. Those cancer patients who are interested are invited to try it as well.

Simonton and his treatment of cancer victims have been criticized for years for a particular type of imagery exercise. By thinking positive images, patients are supposed to be able to enhance the potency of their immune systems. The technique was developed by Carl Simonton, Stephanie Matthews-Simonton, and psychologist Jeanne Achterberg-Lawlis of the University of Texas Health Science Center. Patients are asked first to relax and then envision, in some symbolic manner, the immune system attacking the cancer.

Every set of images should have certain characteristics: the cancer cells should be weak and confused; any treatment visualized should be strong and powerful; the images representing the white blood cells should be vast in number and aggressive in their actions; the cancer cells should be envisioned as being flushed from the body.

The specifics of the images depend on the patient's own ingenuity. Patients have variously envisioned the cancer cells as small, frightened fish and white cells as voracious sharks, or as small, slow-moving creatures ridden down by an army of white knight lymphocytes.

The advantages of the technique, say its proponents, are that it is nontoxic, and that it involves the patient in dealing with the disease directly, rather than maintaining the role of the spectator as the technology of medicine does. And at the very least it improves the quality of the patient's life.

The Simonton method has several shortcomings. Most basic is the difference between their attitudes and those of psychoneuroimmunologists. The science of PNI, too, is fascinated with "healing" images, but at present it is exploring them as a purely experimental method.

Robert Ader outlined the problems when he said, "It's one thing to argue about whether imagery works at all; a second issue to demonstrate that imagery in fact changes immune function; and still a third to say that those particular changes in immune function have any bearing whatsoever on the disease process for which the imagery was introduced in the first place. Don't misunderstand me," he cautioned, "it's a perfectly legitimate hypothesis. But we're short of data to prove that."

In defense of his method, Simonton has said that patients of his who had severe cancers had longer survival times than similar patients who had not participated in the program. Generally, Simonton and Matthews-Simonton have claimed that their cancer patients live twice as long as typical cases mentioned in the cancer literature.

Simonton alludes to one pilot study of a group of his breast cancer patients who lived an average 38.5 months as compared to the average survival time of patients with similar cancers, an average of only 29 months. Usually, research involves a control group, individuals who do not get the drug or the therapy tested; those controls are the same age and sex as those getting the treatment. To eliminate as many variables as possible, researchers try to match for other factors as well. Since Simonton matched his specific cases only against general health statistics, his pilot study makes an interesting, but scientifically weak, point. Comparing real people to statistical averages (sometimes called *historical controls* because they are examples taken from medical history) does not produce persuasive data; it is the weakest form of controlled experiment. The keys to any valid experiment are appropriate controls. The burden of demonstrating that the control group is appropriate falls on the researcher.

Another contaminating factor in Simonton's research is the kind of cancer patient who seeks out his program and programs like his. They are not typical cancer patients. Psychologist Barrie Cassileth says that they tend to be a self-selected group: well educated, intelligent, and certainly not average. Michael Lerner also found that many of the people who seek out these alternative therapies are highly committed individuals, who are "healthy" in the sense of being well-adjusted and who tend to be survivors.

Simonton's patients may survive longer because they are in better physical, and fiscal, shape to begin with. They tend to be mostly white, middle-class (average income around $32,000), and able to have their health insurance underwrite at least some of the therapy. Those who make the trip to California, although considered to be suffering from advanced cancer, are relatively healthy. They would have to be to make the long journey and to live comfortably away from their doctors and treatment for five days.

That they can take the money and time for the Simonton technique indicates that these patients are supermotivated to get well. Probably, therefore, fewer patients depressed by their disease state are included among the individuals who visit the center. This point in itself is important since, as some research suggests, depression may be a risk factor for the progression of disease.

For some cancer patients, the proposition that they had some responsibility for the onset of the disease and, conversely, could have some control over its cure might engender hope. No doubt there is a life-affirming quality to facing a terrifying disease such as cancer. But this proposition has a dark side.

It involves the quandary that psychoneuroimmunologists call the "double-edged sword." Giving individuals the power to cure their disease gives them the opportunity to fail. This is not for everyone. And feelings of guilt may be stimulated when a cancer patient is convinced that the cause and cure of the disease is within reach—with the "right attitude." By putting the individual in charge of fighting cancer, the holistic practitioner relinquishes responsibility for treatment of the patient. Should that treatment fail, the patient may not see it as the failure of a medicine, or a technology, but of his own spirit.

Writer John Tirman, who survived testicular cancer, analyzed the feeling from a cancer patient's viewpoint:

> The conviction that you can take responsibility for defeating your disease, survive through sheer will and discipline, is undeniably admirable. And that élan must surely turn the tide in some cases. There is a flip side to that sentiment, however, a kind of self-importance. These are the victims who accept a different kind of responsibility for their disease—they believe that they *caused* the illness.

"I toyed with that attitude," he admits. But he rejected it: "The self-indulgence of believing that I caused my disease by emotional distress or a sloppy life—by not having my 'act together'—is like saying that people are poor because they're stupid and lazy." In the end he reduces the situation to one brutal fact of life: "that, at times, completely impersonal forces bludgeon you, that circumstances overwhelm you, that riding it out is the only course available."

This holistic predilection for encouraging the patient to accept this kind of responsibility can be a modern Calvinism. The worse sin is to feel that your life is not under your control; even the burden of self-blame is preferable to a feeling of helplessness.

Certainly part of the allure of the holistic approach is that it offers a more benign alternative to the horrifying prospects of chemotherapy, radiotherapy, and surgery. Because cancer is a disease that medicine can control with mixed effectiveness, some individuals respond to it, not surprisingly, by feeling helpless, hopeless, and severely depressed, notes Dr. Jimmie Holland, Chief of the Psychiatry Service at Memorial Sloan-Kettering Cancer Center. These people often crave some way of reasserting control; Holland characterizes psychobiological approaches, like the Simontons', in this way.

Holland has herself seen casualties among individuals who tried these alternative therapies. The individual may feel better at first: "There is little doubt that a patient's sense of well-being improves once the patient feels that he or she has reestablished a degree of control using a treatment that is touted as naturalistic and innocuous," Holland has said. She has also seen the psychological devastation that results when that sense of well-being fades, when the cancer recurs or spreads. Although the treatment may be "natural," it is not, in her opinion, innocuous.

"The patient who already feels guilty for delaying seeking treatment, or who is vulnerable to self-doubt and depression, may become more upset. There is too much chance of increasing the patient's sense of personal failure," she warns. "Coupled with the high fees and lack of follow-up, these treatments constitute a greater psychological hazard than is usually recognized."

Simonton and those who use his method have, of course, heard about the guilt backlash problem many times. They insist that their goal is not to place an excessive burden on the patient. "That's not what we do," objected one member of the Cancer Support and Education Center, which uses the Simonton technique. "We ask the patient to describe anything—any kind of life crisis—that could have contributed to his illness. It doesn't mean the patient made himself ill, but that he was under an enormous amount of stress and that stress is what caused the illness. And that is how we present it."

Psychologist Jean Achterberg-Lawlis agrees that there is guilt but also thinks that the guilt is part of the process of confronting responsibility. "Everyone who deals with psychology deals with that [guilt]," she says. "I don't care if it's cancer or what. When people take responsibility for their actions, they go through a period of having to blame themselves. A good therapist can deal with that. A poor therapist can't."

Simonton has tried to adjust his therapy to prevent the guilt that it sometimes causes. Now dominating his therapy is his two-year health plan, a combination of dietary advice and attitude change. He tries to encourage hopeful feelings by helping cancer patients set easy-to-attain, low-level goals to relieve some of the burden of guilt. For example, when patients propose to meditate every day, Simonton suggests that they meditate two times a week instead, to avoid disappointment. In the same spirit, Simonton gives his firewalking demonstrations—walking across a fifteen-foot-long bed of live coals in his bare feet—as a dramatic demonstration of capabilities the individual has. (At each demonstration, at least one or two cancer patients try a walk as well.) This procedure is geared to stimulate hope and hopefulness, with the intention that these emotions will have an impact on the patient's disease and quality of life.

Another element of Simonton's revised program is helping patients to confront the fear of death. The reason for this goal is that many patients do not survive for the full two years. He and his staff spend part of a day exploring that worry as well as the recurrence of cancer. One result of confronting fear, rather than ignoring it, says Simonton, is that his present patients seem to experience less guilt than those who try to battle the disease using only imagery.

Even with the changes, some shortcomings in Simonton's method remain. It is based on ideas that have yet to be proved, as became evident in the middle of 1985. At that time a research team led by Barrie Cassileth assembled a list of attitudes that other research had suggested might be useful for predicting the lifespans of cancer patients. Cassileth and her colleagues then interviewed a group of 359 patients having advanced cancer, asking about their feelings of helplessness and hopelessness, their job satisfaction, their general satisfaction with life, and social support they received from family and acquaintances.

Over the course of three and a half years the team analyzed the medical progress of the patients, 204 of whom had advanced cancer, to find a relationship between the patients' attitudes and either their survival rate or the rate at which their cancers recurred. The researchers reached two conclusions: first, none of these psychosocial factors had any value in predicting longevity; second, none of those factors was useful for predicting recurrence of cancer. Like so many other researchers, Cassileth wanted to remind the public that these theories have not been proved and are not yet at the point where they can be considered valuable medical therapies.

As she explained it to one interviewer:

There is a danger to the notion, the yet unproven notion, that one's mind can affect something as biologically overwhelming as an advanced malignant disease. The danger is that if patients buy into the idea that if they only think the right way they will cure their cancers and, in some instances, they fail to be cured, they then assume a burden of guilt and blame for having failed to cure themselves. . . . Unfortunately I have seen this happen on many occasions with patients who feel that it is their responsibility alone to cure themselves.

Another, more subtle objection to putting too much responsibility for disease management on the patient is that it preempts the duties of the doctor. A point not emphasized in medical school is that physicians serve a richly symbolic as well as scientific function. The doctor should understand and tolerate the patient's blame when treatment fails. All too frequently the doctor blames the patient: "The patient *failed* the course of chemotherapy" is a remark commonly made. There are times when people need someone to take the responsibility from them, when they need to have a failed healer. At those times doctors must be prepared to accept a patient's anger. As one doctor who worked with many terminal patients put it: "The doctor is responsible. The patient's dying is his failure."

A well-known phenomenon among oncologists is that a patient who suffers a recurrence of cancer occasionally fires the first oncologist and finds another. Even when the new physician uses practically the same techniques, the cancer patient needs to blame someone. Physicians who recognize this phenomenon can help patients handle their feelings, rather than simply changing doctors to no good purpose.

The failed healer has little role in the holistic world, where there is not much room for failure. When the patient becomes the healer, failure to self-cure is too often attributed to the patient's inability to want to be well. In the end the one trait that will prevent holism from joining scientific medicine is its tragic flaw: its inflexible belief that it is the one true medicine.

In the spirit of holism but much more scientific and useful is the new discipline of behavioral medicine, the clinical expression of PNI. In the history of modern medicine it represents what could be considered the third revolution. The first, the *surgical revolution,* appeared with the introduction of ether anesthesia into the operating room in 1846. Anesthesia allowed physicians to enter the body to repair and correct ailments they were once helpless to fix. With the introduction of penicillin in 1941 came the *chemical revolution:* miracle drugs gave doctors what were considered at that time to be the ultimate weapons against infectious diseases. After a while it became evident that chemicals could not work certain miracles. In the 1960s the time was right for another change, the *behavioral revolution.*

Traditional psychosomatic medicine with its heavily psychoanalytic approach was unable to fulfill its promise. Psychoanalytic therapies proved to have limited usefulness in the treatment of the classic "Holy Seven" psychosomatic illnesses. The recognition of psychological components in other ailments not generally considered psychosomatic blurred the distinction between psychosomatic and "nonpsychosomatic" diseases.

The new awareness of these aspects of wellness was synthesized in behavioral medicine, which officially became a new discipline in a 1977 conference at Yale University. There psychologists, psychiatrists, and specialists of all kinds convened to discuss how they could help medicine incorporate into modern clinical practice the insight that people could do more to control the state of their health.

The conference generated a new model for healing. Behavioral medicine expert and psychologist Ovid Pomerleau of the University of Connecticut explains that four conditions are intrinsic to therapeutic programs that could be considered behavioral: trying to change a behavioral (such as the circumstances surrounding asthma attacks) or physiological response (change in the glucose of a diabetic) that is in itself a health problem; changing the ways health care providers work by improving their methods of caring for the sick (for example, by teaching the value of paying attention to the patient or by touching or listening); trying to improve compliance to a given treatment; and stepping in to change behaviors or responses (such as smoking) that are risk factors.

This new brand of medicine is multidisciplined and emphasizes the individual's active role in maintaining health and preventing illness. It is based on the premise that the true power of healing resides in the patient *as much as* the doctor. Although this approach involves the patient in the treatment, it does not transfer the full burden of healing to the patient nor does it espouse one therapy as *the* way to health.

Behavioral medicine is not based on any one system of healing; rather, it is an inspirational, eclectic attitude, a spirit that has come to perfuse twentieth-century medicine. Using the experimental, nondogmatic approach of behavioral medicine, PNI researchers have learned to use the techniques and therapies suggested by a broad mix of scientific experts: clinical psychologists, epidemiologists, experimental psychologists, medical anthropologists, physiologists, psychiatrists, and sociologists. (In fact, because it includes the interaction of behavior and immunology, PNI is sometimes referred to as behavioral immunology.)

The result of all these experts' efforts is not one therapy but a collection of them. Each one applies the knowledge and insights gleaned from their research and clinical practice. Each one has its own unique therapeutic value. Although several will be recognized as those often used by holistic practitioners, there is a difference in the way they are used. First, no PNI researcher will claim any one of these methods is "the answer," the ultimate PNI prescription. If the research to date has proven anything, it is that there are no simple answers.

That leads to our second point: each of these is just a part of a larger and more complex program of therapies constantly evolving from psychoneuroimmunological research and discoveries. Just as in pharmacology no one medicine works for everyone, no one PNI therapy is universally beneficial. And so the following elements of the PNI prescription are offered with the understanding that none of them is best, and that they have produced some encouraging results for the treatment of certain conditions and show promise for the future.

Invariably every behavioral treatment strategy includes in its plan some form of relaxation technique to counter the erosive effects of stress. At the very least the relaxation exercise helps clear the mind of distractions and lets the person doing the exercise feel good for a brief period of time. Further, the research data related to states of mind and body suggest that relaxation may even defuse some of the immunosuppressing effects of stress.

As yet, no relaxation method is demonstrably superior to others. Some, such as biofeedback, use biomedical equipment and audio signals to inform individuals that they have reached a plateau of relaxation. Others require only a few minutes a day and a little willpower.

Progressive Relaxation

In terms of pure body relaxation and simplicity, one very popular method is progressive muscle relaxation, sometimes called the *Jacobson Technique* after the University of Chicago researcher, Edmund Jacobson, who developed it in the 1930s. It is used in sleep laboratories to help insomniacs to relax, in behavioral medicine programs to help cardiac patients soften their Type A behavior, and in a variety of stress-management programs.

First, an individual finds a quiet place to sit. Then, starting with the feet and lower legs, the person progressively tenses and then relaxes the distinct muscle groups of the body, first tensing the left hand and then the right hand at the same time. Next, the following are tensed and then relaxed: both forearms, the upper arms, the forehead, both eyes, the nose, both cheeks and mouth, neck, chest, back, abdomen, upper legs, calves, and feet. Each muscle group is tensed for a slow count of ten seconds. The point is to concentrate on the muscles as they unclench, to savor the relaxing sensations that flow from them.

This method is easy to learn, requires no special equipment, and can be done almost anywhere. It uses the body's own sensations to provide the relaxing feeling, and feedback is immediate and noticeable.

Autogenic Training

Autogenic training (AT) is a system of "passive concentration" developed around the turn of the century by the German psychotherapist Johannes Schultz. It relies on a kind of self-hypnosis in which the practitioner repeats verbal formulae organized into six groups of exercises. The formulae are related to different sensations in the body. Using "passive" concentration, the practitioner senses changes within the body that follow repetition of the verbal messages. The individual does not try to direct the changes; after a while, the body responds to them. A ritual called the *autogenic formulae* uses specific combinations of phrases to obtain certain effects.

First is "My right arm is heavy," which is repeated for all the limbs, with "My ——— is warm." That is followed by concentrating on the heartbeat: "Heartbeat calm and regular." Then the practitioner emphasizes the breath: "It breathes me," ending with "My forehead is cool."

Like progressive relaxation, autogenic training calms the mind and body. It is very effective, but one of its drawbacks is that according to its master practitioners learning how to do the exercises so that they are effective requires four to ten months of practice.

Biofeedback

Similar in effect but more complicated in application is biofeedback. The procedure uses electronic equipment that detects subtle changes in a person's body via sensors attached to the scalp or fingertips, for example. The machine gives off one type of signal, usually a tone or light, when the body is relaxing and another when it is tensing. The machine reads these states of tension or relaxation when the brain begins to generate more alpha waves or, for other equipment, when the galvanic skin response, the electrical conductivity of the skin, changes.

Biofeedback helps individuals to learn to control or change those electronic signals to attain an optimal state of relaxation. Biofeedback allows people to achieve what were once considered yogic feats—slowing the heartbeat, redirecting the circulation—by listening to or watching the biofeedback signal, observing the body in action. The principal advantage this technique has over other relaxation methods is that before their very eyes (or ears) patients get persuasive evidence of the mind-body relationship.

Biofeedback takes the real but sometimes unnoticed turmoil the body experiences and makes it more detectable. It has been used to treat a variety of ailments. Dr. George Fuller-von Bozzay of the Biofeedback Institute of San Francisco cites a case in which a five-year-old girl who had severe asthma attacks benefited from bio-feedback techniques.

The small child learned to make herself "quiet inside" by playing with a biofeedback machine that measured her skin temperature. She could raise or lower her hand temperature at will within fifteen minutes of trying. She was able to transfer her skills to her breathing by, for example, thinking of her chest as a balloon that would fill up and then pushing the air out. Before the biofeedback training, she was spending roughly one week a month in the intensive care ward, recovering from asthma attacks. After treatment she had gone two years, at last record, without a severe attack.

Relaxation Response

One of the simplest of all relaxation techniques, the easiest to learn and easiest to practice, is the method that evokes the *relaxation response* conceived by Harvard Medical School cardiologist Dr. Herbert Benson. In the late 1960s he had been studying monkeys to find a connection between the animals' behavior and their blood pressure. Practitioners of Transcendental Meditation (TM) told him they could lower their blood pressure without drugs whenever they wished. "Why investigate anything so far out as meditation?" he was to recall years later.

But the advocates of TM persisted, and Benson changed his mind, influenced by a paper published in *Science* magazine, "Physiological Effects of Transcendental Meditation" by Keith Wallace, a young Ph.D. candidate in physiology at the University of California. Wallace was an experienced meditator and had decided to use his skills as a scientist to measure effects on the bodies of people who were meditating. Their blood pressure decreased; oxygen consumption dropped; brain waves resembled those of people in the relaxed alpha-wave state recorded by biofeedback.

When Wallace came to work with Benson at Harvard Medical

School's Thorndike Laboratory, he and Benson found that the people practicing Zen or yoga exercises were able to achieve many of the same effects. Progressive relaxation and autogenic training had the same results. Benson also noted that when they prayed or meditated, deeply religious people, especially mystics, settled into an identical soothing state of mind.

After more research, he and his fellow scientists found that all these methods had four basic features in common.

- Each was performed in a quiet place: a cool, shaded room; a temple, church, or chapel.

- Each had an object of concentration: a symbol or single sound like the famous *Om* to focus on.

- Each practitioner assumed a comfortable position.

- Most importantly, to perform the exercise successfully, individuals assumed a passive attitude, a willingness to let thoughts pass through the mind without dwelling on any one. They were not to worry whether they were performing the exercise correctly or well. The resulting exercise could summon forth Benson's *relaxation response,* a becalming state of body and spirit.

Benson theorizes that the relaxation response, in its various forms, operates through the hypothalamus, which is important in the nervous system's influence over the immune system. He bases his theory on work by Swiss Nobel Laureate Dr. Walter Hess on the brains of cats. When Hess stimulated one section of the hypothalamus with small pulses of electricity he obtained a trophotropic response, the feline equivalent of the relaxation response. The animal was placid and had some of the same body patterns—lowered blood pressure, relaxed muscles—that the TM and relaxation response groups had.

Out of these insights came the relaxation response formula (see Books section in Appendix B), which, in the years since its introduction, has become a potent tool of behavioral medicine. At Boston's Beth Israel Hospital where Benson directs the Division of Behavioral Medicine, he has incorporated his relaxation response into two programs—one for patients with hypertension, and the other the

Mind/Body Group (described in Chapter Six)—for individuals having many kinds of ailments from migraine headaches to diabetes.

Once criticized for his involvement in a scientific fad, Benson is now recognized as a pioneer of behavioral medicine. His method has withstood the test of a decade of use and is considered by some to be the best of the relaxation exercises. It requires no elaborate rituals or beliefs and is simple and easy to learn. When he first began to test it, Benson recruited from the Boston area people who had never used any relaxation techniques and simply handed them a sheet of instructions. Within a few minutes they were using less oxygen as they practiced, a sign of deep relaxation.

Research with the relaxation response has legitimized with scientific evidence the mind's real, physical effect on the body, making it acceptable for people to believe that they can have control over their health.

EXERCISE

We still know little about the potential effect of a steady regimen of exercise on individuals, except that it makes them feel good and prevents heart disease. Everyone "knows" good exercise habits have specific health benefits, including protection against cardiovascular disease, retardation of the aging process, and weight control through burning up calories. But in the past few years evidence has indicated that other, more subtle benefits result. Exercise is, therefore, becoming an important component of behavioral medicine.

One reason is that exercise has psychological benefit. A weekly ritual of working out can modify some personality characteristics slightly. One is reduction of tension. Sports medicine expert Dr. Herbert DeVries has found that muscle tension decreases in people after a short (five- to thirty-minute) session of light exercise. Jogging, cycling, or even walking at 30 to 60 percent of maximum heartbeat capacity can act as a mild anxiety reducer and antidepressant.

To the PNI researcher the latter finding is significant, especially since depression is associated with a weakened immune system. Therefore, exercise is not only a natural antidepressant but, if psychoneuroimmunological evidence is correct, it may provide a kind of immunological insurance, especially for individuals susceptible to depression.

Evidence also suggests that exercise triggers specific biochemicals, the most famous of which are the endorphins, the body's natural opiates. According to University of New Mexico sports medicine specialist Dr. Otto Appenzeller, these body chemicals give the boost to the runner/swimmer/cyclist's high and may be the chemical source of the antidepressant effect of a good workout. Once set loose, these opiates linger in the body long after the exercise is finished. For example, blood samples taken from a group of men who had just finished a grueling twenty-seven-mile run up a mountain showed that high levels of endorphins were still in their bodies two hours after the race.

Another side effect of exercise may be to enhance the immune system's germ-fighting potential. During and after a heavy workout an athlete may have a slight fever: the more active the exercise, the higher the temperature rise, up to three degrees above normal. Someone who runs a brisk eight-minute mile experiences a three-degree boost, whereas someone playing a less active sport such as baseball has only a slight temperature rise. This phenomenon is similar to a bodily response to infection called an *acute-phase immune response,* which, physiologists think, slows the reproduction of bacteria and viruses.

Physiologists knew about this phenomenon for years, but no one was able to explain why it happened. University of Michigan physiologist Joseph Cannon suspects that one of the reasons for the temperature climb is a substance called *endogenous pyrogen,* also known as *interleukin-1,* produced by the immune system's macrophage cells. The substance travels in the bloodstream to the brain's temperature control center. There it trips a signal to raise the body's temperature. The T- and B-cells grow slightly more rapidly at a higher body temperature. Interleukin-1 also breaks down muscle protein into raw material the immune system uses to fight infection. (For this reason, fever is often accompanied by an achy feeling.) Cannon and his coresearcher Matthew Kluger speculate that these same endogenous pyrogens are released during exercise.

To test their hypothesis, they took two blood samples from subjects: the first immediately before they began exercising and the second after each person had pedaled for an hour on an exercycle.

Both samples were injected into rats. The preexercise blood samples caused no noticeable reaction, but the postexercise blood produced fever, a higher white blood cell count, and a drop of zinc and iron levels in the blood—typical acute immune responses. Although yet to be proved, Cannon's guess is that the body uses this response as a primitive protective mechanism, one that evolved from more primitive days when people ran, not for exercise, but to escape danger. Their bodies were able to turn on the pyrogen system to prepare for any injuries that might occur.

THE RETURN OF FRANZ MESMER

Not every new therapy in psychoimmunology is really new. Some excellent techniques have existed for centuries, often forgotten. More and more we see the wisdom in Mark Twain's observation that "the ancients have stolen all our best ideas." An old procedure that has generated lively new interest was discovered by an eighteenth-century Viennese doctor named Franz Mesmer. Mesmer was an upper-class physician who, until 1774, lived a comfortable life, unremarkable except for his socializing with some of the greatest classical musicians of his era: Glück, Haydn, Mozart.

On July 28, 1774, Mesmer's life was transformed when he tried out a new therapy called *magnetism* on a patient. A female patient had been especially resistant to standard treatments, so he decided to attempt "magnetic therapy," as it was called. Using three specially designed magnets, he placed one on her stomach and one on each of her legs. The woman claimed to feel the flow of a fluid coursing through her body. In a matter of hours she felt dramatically better. Mesmer theorized that the magnets had stirred up a vital fluid he named *animal magnetism.* Her recovery was so dramatic that Mesmer was convinced he had a true panacea, a cure for every disease.

From then, he dedicated himself to testing the potential of the amazing force. He used no medicines other than "magnetized" water or a bathtub full of iron filings. In time he realized that the real power of healing lay not in the magnets, but in him. So he threw them away and used an apparently genuinely charismatic gift of healing to treat those brought to him. Mesmer seemed able to cure people by the force of his personality. He could stare into the eyes of a patient, pass his hands over the afflicted parts of the body, and produce wondrous results.

For a few years Mesmer's name was on everyone's lips. In Paris he had several influential disciples, among them the Marquis de Lafayette and a physician in the king's court. But by 1785, nine years after he had made his magnetic discovery, his contemporaries in medicine considered him a threat, and gradually Mesmer and his fantastic powers were discredited. He was arrested and stood trial as a quack. The remainder of his life he spent in obscurity.

The movement of Mesmerism lived on, becoming immensely popular in France, Germany, and eventually in England. The work of a British doctor, James Braid, who could "mesmerize" some people by asking them to stare at a shiny object helped to legitimize it. Braid rejected the Mesmerist explanation that this effect was the result of animal magnetism, and he renamed the technique *hypnosis,* from a Greek root word meaning "sleep." But after this spasm of scientific legitimacy, Mesmerism degenerated into a kind of cult, and hypnotism itself became little more than a music hall trick.

Interest in it was revived by the brilliant nineteenth-century French neurologist, Jean-Martin Charcot, whose work inspired Sigmund Freud. In the early days of psychotherapy, Freud used hypnotism as a means of exploring the subconscious. He moved on to other methods, but hypnosis came to be identified more with psychotherapy and less with medicine. Some of its medical potency faded from memory.

Today, a more scientific brand of Franz Mesmer's magnetism prevails in the hospital and doctor's office. Over the years, skilled hypnotists have been using hypnotic trances with varying degrees of success for treating migraine headaches, asthma, and circulatory problems. Some suggest that more subtle controls could be exerted over more intricate processes of the body.

The most dramatic scientific evidence of the potential of hypnosis has come from experts working with burns, both real and illusory. According to hypnosis specialist Theodore X. Barber of Cushing Hospital in Framingham, Massachusetts, hypnotists have been able to produce the sensation, even the physical mark, of burns. He once hypnotized a group of nurses and told them their hands were being splashed with scalding grease. One nurse developed a skin inflammation, which appeared in the identical spot where she had actually burned her hand a few years before. Another hypnotist laid a cool copper disk on the skin of a hypnotized woman. After he told her that it was a red-hot coin, she shrieked with pain, and a few hours later a blister the precise diameter of the coin appeared on her skin.[1]

To a psychoneuroimmunologist the hypnosis experiments that are especially tantalizing are those that seem to generate a reaction from the immune system. Some of the most intriguing work has been done with the common wart. As writer-physician Lewis Thomas indicates, "warts can be ordered off the skin by hypnotic suggestion."

The life and death of warts has fascinated psychoneuroimmunologists for years for several reasons. They have a known medical cause: a virus. As the product of enemy microbes, warts invite battle with the immune system. Sometimes the immune system wins a skirmish; sometimes it loses, as the persistence of a wart testifies. Still, it is unclear why they disappear when they do.

Sometimes the medicine that eliminates warts is no stronger than a thought. Curing warts by conviction has a long history in folklore as well as in medicine. Mark Twain wrote about it in *Tom Sawyer* in an incident in which Huckleberry Finn shares his prescription with Tom:

> You got to go all by yourself to the middle of the woods where you know there's a spunk-water stump, and just as it's midnight you back up against the stump and jam your hand in and say:
> "Barley-corn, Barley-corn, Injun-meal shorts
> Spunk-water, Spunk-water, swaller these warts."

And in Huckleberry Finn's bean prescription:

> You take and split the bean, and cut the wart so as to get some blood, and then you put the blood on one piece of the bean and take and dig a hole and bury it 'bout midnight at the crossroads in the dark of the moon, and then you burn up the rest of the bean. You see that piece that's got the blood on it will keep drawing and drawing, trying to fetch the other piece to it, and so that helps the blood to draw the wart, and pretty soon off she comes.

Even in the world of science, Theodore X. Barber says that physicians have used more sophisticated versions of the same approach. During the 1920s Dr. Bruno Bloch was a world-famous wart specialist in Zurich. The secret of his success was a "wart-killing machine," a wonderful apparatus that emitted an impressive noise, glittered with flashing lights, and—Bloch told his patients—beamed lethal antiwart rays at the offending growth. Patients were cured by the dozens. Dr. Bloch's gadget in fact had all the curing powers of Huck Finn's beans. The apparatus was a totally useless electronic creation with a motor inside that whirred and whirred and did little else. Somehow in the belief in Dr. Bloch's gadget the true medicine lay.

Over the years dozens of experimenters have tried to produce the same results with warts and other problems by using hypnosis. One who has become an experienced hypnotherapist is clinical psychologist Ted Grossbart. For years he has been using a combination of psychotherapy, hypnosis, self-hypnosis, and imagery to help patients with persistent and disfiguring skin disorders.

The largest organ in the human body, skin is particularly susceptible to ailments having a psychological component. It is Grossbart's thesis that emotions play havoc with skin diseases.

"The two most common human agonies that provide the underlying fuel for skin diseases are anger and loss of love," he says: the face of an angry person becomes flushed and red; someone in love may blush to get attention and affection. "In people who are looking for compassion that hasn't been there and for whatever reason have been unable to find it or ask for it, their skin takes over the task of looking for love or expressing the anger." By exposing these buried emotional themes and helping a person deal with them, Grossbart has been trying to defuse the dermatological time bombs. Over the past few years he has treated eczema, hives, warts, and genital herpes.

Grossbart has been using a combination of hypnosis and relaxation exercises, whose purpose is to help a patient to shift attention from the disease, to use imagery to change physiological conditions, and to understand the meaning of the symptoms.

Grossbart's applications of these principles vary from one person to another. Typically he tries to find out which sensations and images make a patient's skin feel better. Then he tries to help the patient mentally recreate that ideal environment. For a patient with a maddening rash on his feet the technique might be fantasizing an ankle-deep stroll through the icy waters of a mountain brook. For another, it might be imagining baking in the hot sun at a beach. One person imagined himself sitting in front of an open hearth with a roaring fire, feet propped up and being warmed. (The patient attained such proficiency that he could raise the temperature of his toes by about five degrees.)

Grossbart's goal is to heighten the emotional sensitivity of his patients to make them aware of the events within them: in Grossbart's words, "to listen to their skin." The next step is to realize what these skin ailments are telling the victims and to "change their head or their heart" to take control and consciously direct this anger and frustrated love away from a self-destructive course and redirect those energies in a more constructive way.

One of Grossbart's patients was a carpenter in his late twenties whose hands were so encrusted with warts that they were grotesque ("It was really quite grim," says Grossbart. "It looked like one of those photos you see of lepers"). A hypnotic trance would alleviate some of the pain, but try as he might, the young man could not make the warts disappear.

Grossbart then decided to shift tactics slightly. He asked the man to try imaging, to conjure up an imaginary work crew whose job was dismantling the layers of warts that encrusted his hands. The carpenter actually talked aloud to the crew about what they were to do. In the midst of one of these conversations, he let slip an important piece of information: one of the imaginary crew members pointed out that once all the warts were removed, the young man would have to deal with his real problem, shyness with women.

Hearing this, Grossbart made a deal with the man and his crew. Since getting rid of the warts was of prime importance, he suggested that the crew do that first. Later he and the carpenter could discuss his shyness problem. "Within about three weeks this incredible crop of warts vanished," Grossbart recalls, himself impressed.

If hypnosis can perform such feats for comparatively mild medical ailments such as warts, what can it do for more serious medical conditions? According to some experts, hypnosis has a promising future in treating severely burned victims. When a Louisiana factory worker had a nightmarish industrial accident (he slipped and stepped into a pool of molten aluminum), he was rushed to the local hospital. The first forty-eight hours after a burn are especially critical; during that period burn victims are in danger of shock, or their immune system is so battered they can succumb to infections.

When the man was admitted for treatment, Dr. Dabney Edwin, professor of surgery and psychiatry at Tulane University, hypnotized him. Edwin is among a small group of physicians who use hypnosis to treat severe burn victims. After producing a trance, Edwin began telling the patient that his seared leg was beginning to feel cool and comfortable. To his doctors' surprise, the man recovered from a potentially grave, disfiguring accident with no serious infections, no complications, and no scar tissue.

Hypnotizing a patient within hours of an injury, says Edwin, can have a significant effect on the speed and completeness of recovery. One of the first procedures he performs for burn victims is making a hypnotic suggestion that they will feel a cooling sensation in the burned area. The result is more than the illusion of soothing comfort. This procedure minimizes damage and inflammation so well that Edwin has seen patients who would have ordinarily required skin grafts heal without them.

At the Alta Bates Hospital's burn center in Berkeley, California, burn center director Dr. Jerold Kaplan, too, has been using hypnosis. Kaplan takes patients with burns on both sides of their bodies and, after hypnotizing them, asks them to try to make the temperature of one side higher than that on the other. The patients were able to raise their temperatures by as much as 4°C; in addition, the side with the temperature increase healed faster than the unwarmed side.

What is the source of this power? No one is sure. Psychiatrist Owen Surman of Massachusetts General Hospital's Department of Psychiatry received an indication during some hypnosis work of his own. In one memorable and particularly satisfying case, he treated a Boston police officer who had plantar warts—warts on the soles of his feet—that were so painful the man could barely walk. When the officer first consulted Surman, he was receiving payments for a total disability. Standard medical treatments had little effect; only the suggestion under hypnosis that the warts were shrinking seemed to help.

Curious about the processes occurring inside the man during these sessions, Surman asked the policeman to allow his brain to be monitored by a positron emission transaxial tomography (PETT) scan, essentially an in-depth three-dimensional X ray, while he was in a hypnotic trance. The scan showed a distinct activity in the frontal lobes of his brain, suggesting to Surman that whatever directives were sent to the immune system were originating in that region. It occurred in only one case, Surman cautions, but adds hopefully, "it is tempting to think of a cure for warts stored somewhere in the frontal lobes."

Also present in the frontal lobes may be the power some individuals have to withstand pain and alter basic physical reactions. The best recent example of this phenomenon is the self-improvement craze of firewalking. With only a few hours of instruction, average, nonmystical people have learned to walk across eight-, ten-, twenty-, even forty-foot beds of hot coals incandescently glowing at about 1200°F. Those who offer firewalking instruction frequently claim that the combination of their self-improvement courses and the experience of literally walking on fire can cause a profound transformation of the psyche. By being able to overcome the fear of fire and pain and to walk on the coals, the logic goes, a person gains the confidence to attempt any goal.

Whether or not walking twelve feet through coals can work this kind of inner transformation is open to question; that thousands of people can and have taken firewalks is not. Most not only felt no pain, but did not suffer so much as a blister.

Sceptics offer various explanations. Some invoke a phenomenon of physics called the *Leidenfrost effect:* a thin layer of moisture, for example, saliva used to moisten the fingers before pinching out a candle flame, insulates the skin from the flame with a boundary of steam. In firewalking training, perspiration or a layer of water on the skin (participants walk through wet grass before the firewalk) may provide such a protective layer.

Another possible explanation is offered by UCLA physicist Bernard Leikin: that the coals in the fire, though red-hot, are not dense and therefore are poor conductors of heat. A foot may conceivably step on a hot coal and move on before an appreciable amount of heat is transferred, and a burn results.

As for the inner experience of the firewalk, alternative medicine specialist Dr. Andrew Weil has watched firewalks and has taken a few himself, at times developing a few blisters for his adventurousness. He believes that the Leidenfrost effect simply does not explain the entire phenomenon. For example, he and other observers have noticed that firewalkers appear to enter into a quasi-hypnotic trance as they cross the coals, sometimes chanting firewalk mantras ("Cool Moss" is a favorite) as they stroll. "There is no question in my mind that a person's mental state is the crucial variable," Weil states. "To experience no heat and no inflammation is not explainable in mechanistic terms. My intuitive sense says that the nervous system is functioning in a different way than is usual. That has something to do with being in a state of total relaxation and non-defensiveness." In fact, Weil adds that one of his more successful walks—over forty feet of live coals—occurred when he felt that he had slipped into a kind of altered state, one that may have protected him from the ravages of the fire.

Entrancing the Immune System

Given the feats humans have accomplished through hypnosis, it is only natural that others have wondered how deeply its effects can be felt. At Pennsylvania State University, Howard Hall, a psychologist and hypnotist, has been studying the effects of hypnosis on a cellular level. He explains: "I'm interested in what you can do with hypnosis. Can you alter various biochemicals? Can we alter the immune system?"

Inspired by the work of Carl Simonton, which uses images in an attempt to send immune cells into battle with cancer cells, Hall decided to adapt it for an experiment. He hypnotized twenty healthy people aged twenty-two to eighty-five. (He deliberately chose a broad age spread because the immune systems of elderly persons are typically weaker than those of younger individuals and are said to allow a natural increase of cancer cells.) He taught the group self-hypnosis, telling them to imagine their white blood cells as "strong and powerful sharks" attacking any germ cells roaming their bodies. He took a blood sample before the session and an hour afterward. The group was sent home and told to perform self-hypnosis on their own. Two weeks later, the group returned to Hall's laboratory for a third blood sample.

A select few had a noticeably more active immune response to the test. The younger, that is to say those under fifty, had a significantly higher immune response, as did those rated as highly responsive to hypnotism. Hall has not offered an explanation of these results and is careful to say that his is only a preliminary peek at the immunopotency of hypnosis. The results he has seen have been tantalizing enough to keep him researching the subject. This glimpse of a positive force of the mind in action has led Hall to suggest that using this combination of hypnosis and visualization to enhance the psychology of healing is within the realm of possibility.

THE MIND'S EYE

Hypnosis is one way of focusing the mind's attention. More controversial but equally fascinating is the technique of *mental imagery,* conjuring up pictures in the mind to try to produce a specific effect. With sufficiently vivid mental scenes, many people can produce physical results. Is a unique process at work? How profound are its effects? Are they strong enough to nudge health of an individual in one direction or another?

Most hypnosis specialists consider mental imagery a variant of hypnosis, *autohypnosis.* Apparently no mystical or mysterious element differentiates it from hypnosis. Although it does have a magical sound, imagery is only another version of Franz Mesmer's technique. Obviously, people like Dr. Simonton believe that this technique is a new therapy. Specialists in psychoneuroimmunology are more cautious in their claims for the technique but find it a fertile source of research and speculation.

Imagery does work on some levels. Anyone who is sceptical that images in the mind can influence involuntary body processes should try the following imagery exercise. (It is more effective if someone reads this section aloud to you, or, if that is not possible, if you read it into a tape recorder yourself and play it back. In either case the reader should pause for three or four seconds between sentences.)

Before starting, find a comfortable sitting position in a quiet room. Get settled. Relax. Now listen and let the images take over.

Imagery Exercise*

Imagine yourself in your kitchen.

Look around at the familiar objects in your kitchen: the sink, the stove, the refrigerator.

Open the refrigerator door. Notice the little light comes on. You may even feel a little bit of the cold air.

Look around and find that part of the refrigerator in which you keep lemons. Perhaps it's a drawer.

Take out a lemon. You'll feel the cold of the lemon in the palm of your hand. Close the refrigerator door.

Heft the lemon in your hand and feel its weight.

Squeeze it a little bit. Feel its rubbery consistency.

Examine the skin. Notice the little pores on the surface of the skin.

Notice that the lemon has two little chubby ends.

Put the lemon down and take out your favorite kitchen knife, a nice sharp knife. Cut the lemon in half by the little chubby ends, crosswise.

When you have done that, pick up one half of the lemon and look at the freshly cut surface. Look at the little lemon segments. If you look at it very closely, you'll see little tiny droplets of lemon juice are beginning to form on that surface.

And if you squeeze the lemon just slightly, the drops will begin to coalesce, and you'll now see a sheet of lemon juice on the surface of the lemon.

Lick the lemon across the whole surface and taste the sourness of the lemon juice. It's almost enough to wrinkle up your face.

*Used by courtesy of Erik Peper, Ph.D.

Did you salivate? As a general rule, about half of any group of people respond to these images.

Over the years researchers of all kinds have taken this ability beyond simple matters of making salivary glands function on command. The science of healthful imagery is still very new, but it has tantalized doctors with its potential. One who has been impressed is neuroendocrinologist Nicholas Hall, of the Department of Biochemistry at George Washington University. Thinking back on his participation in the imagery research done with cancer patients at the Washington School of Psychiatry, he remembered in particular one case that involved a man in his mid-sixties, a retired school administrator. As part of the experiment, he kept a meticulous diary describing his feelings about his daily imagery practice sessions. He was enthusiastic about the experiment, going so far as to postpone some chemotherapy treatments so as not to affect the blood samples taken for the study.

Part of Hall's function was to monitor the levels of the hormone thymosin in the man's blood. Thymosin is very important in augmenting the immune response, Hall explained, and its concentrations would provide one indicator of the potency of the man's immune system. Levels were checked against the man's moods and attitudes recorded in his diary.

On days when he felt that the imagery exercises were going well, the man's thymosin levels were high. On days when his diary showed that he was not participating fully in the imaging, his thymosin levels were lower. In the midst of the study, the man's wife died. He wrote in his diary that he had lost interest in the experiment. A blood sample was drawn at the same time. Laboratory tests showed that his thymosin levels were noticeably depressed. The man stopped doing the imagery work; two months later, he died. "The emotional setbacks, coupled with cancer, were too much," Hall says. "In my opinion, he essentially gave up hope."

Experiments such as Hall's raise more questions than they answer. Had the imagery kept the man alive? Did it make any difference at all in his health? Are there, as some claim, powerful, healing images, or ineffectual, even dangerous images? The simple answer is that, despite the beliefs of many advocates of holistic cures, we do not know. From the evidence accumulated so far, it appears that imagery exercises have some effect, but that the specific image does not. There are no inherently healthful images. They are healthful only to the degree that the people using them experience some sort of feeling of well-being or security—the same kind of feeling that accompanies hope of recovery. Since mimicking emotions can cause internal changes, it appears probable that genuine emotions produce subtle alterations in the internal milieu, changes that are not yet known. These alterations in turn could effect subtle changes in the neurochemistry or neurophysiology of the immune system. But stating that the visual images somehow directly marshall the forces of the immune system and that they are literally translated by the brain into brain-to-cell chemical messages would be premature because it would not take into account the complexities of the human system and the realities of sickness.

At this point, we have some sense of the potential benefits and limitations of the various methods discussed so far: biofeedback, the relaxation response, hypnosis, exercise, and imagery. Research evidence justifies some cautious optimism that in addition to the medicines and therapies of the hospital and the clinic, alternative healthful methods may be efficacious.

Individuals have always believed that the mind affects the body; now that belief can be confirmed. Even so, psychoneuroimmunologists do not believe that they are on the verge of discovering Panacea, the cure to end all cures. Any given methodology is just a piece of a very complex and incomplete picture of the potential of medical science. Many holistic believers tend to overlook that point. Although we need a medicine that is more catholic and less technocratic, we must not replace the science of medicine with an all-encompassing belief in Panacea: the human machine is too complicated.

CHAPTER TEN

The New Medicine
and the
Biology of Hope

SEVERAL YEARS AGO, psychiatrist Joel Dimsdale, then at Massachusetts General Hospital, tracked down and interviewed survivors of the Nazi death camps. What was it, Dimsdale wanted to know, that kept them going? What kept them alive?

After studying the interviews, Dimsdale isolated several coping strategies for survival: focusing on the few good experiences one had; trying to master the environment through asserting one's individuality—by observing Jewish holidays, for example; determining to survive for a special purpose; using a numbing process he calls *psychological removal;* having the primal will to live; possessing a group affiliation; and adapting other irregular strategies, such as childlike behavior to elicit sympathy from guards or other inmates, being totally passive, and even accepting the Nazis' attitudes toward them.

But out of all the answers he obtained and all the survival stories he heard, one attitude was echoed in the testimonies of each survivor. The human quality that kept these people alive, he says, was "blind, naked hope." Some people survived by setting goals for themselves. One survivor said that the thought of being reunited with her family kept her going. Others focused on what few pleasant experiences they had in the prison camp—getting an extra scrap of food, enjoying the sun on a spring day.

Among the goals of psychoneuroimmunology is finding the way to summon that hope. Part of its quest is to call forth the biology of hope through an appreciation of the healing powers of the human spirit and a deeper understanding of the intimate neuronal and hormonal bonds between the mind and body. In the remainder of this century and in the one to come, the art of healing and the science of medicine will be transformed by that quest.

We know PNI will rely on the natural pharmacology of attitudes and feelings as well as the tools of technology and the pharmacy of synthetic drugs. The future of medicine is beginning to take shape. Little by little, researchers are analyzing, quantifying, and learning to use resources once considered beyond the reach of scientific inquiry. Today it is possible to measure phenomena that were once immeasurable.

HOPE

What about hope? Can we measure it? Can we invoke it when it is needed? Will it submit to the scales and gauges of science? University of California psychiatrist Dr. Louis Gottschalk believes that he can measure hope by a test called the *content analysis of verbal behavior*. Gottschalk and his colleagues have been asking cancer patients to talk for five minutes about an interesting or dramatic event in their lives. The short talk is tape-recorded, and transcribed, and a trained "rater" evaluates the transcript.

The rater sifts through the transcript, marks key phrases and clauses, and assigns a number, rating them for levels or intensity of a particular emotional state. For anxiety, for example, there are six subtypes, each of which can be recognized and scored for intensity by the experienced rater. By a mathematical formula that measures magnitude of emotion per 100 words, a rater derives a number that indicates a relative score, or measure, of the level of psychological problem a person is experiencing.

The analysis is such that with the transcript of five minutes of talk, a well-trained analyzer can score scripts of human speech "much as biochemical technicians are trained to run various chemical determinations by following prescribed procedures." By scanning for key words, researchers are able to score the intensity of anxiety, hostility, and so forth, through numerical ratings. Gottschalk says that a person trained to read these emotional soliloquies can obtain an objective measurement of states of mind such as anxiety, hostility (directed inward and outward), achievement strivings, and intellectual impairment.

As part of this test, Gottschalk uses a scale that can measure hope in the same way it can measure levels of anxiety and despair. He has used his interview technique with twenty-seven cancer patients receiving radiotherapy at Cincinnati General Hospital and has found that those who had the higher "hope" scores also had higher survival rates.

That result naturally raises the question of whether it will someday be possible to influence those scales, to raise a person's hope quotient. In an effort to activate hope or enhance the feelings that exist, psychiatrist Fred Hencker, a professor of psychiatry at the University of Arkansas, and his colleagues are working on a program to enhance hope in patients slated for heart surgery and kidney transplants. His procedure combines information and human rapport to encourage confidence and hope.

Before an operation patients and their families meet with the surgeon and staff, who explain the upcoming surgical procedures and, just as importantly, give the people involved the opportunity for human contact with one another. After the operation the hospital staff encourages patients to do as much for themselves as they feel able to do. The goal is to induce patients to see themselves not as individuals who are sick so much as individuals who are recovering. "The hope of those in attendance spreads to the patient," explains Dr. Hencker, "augmenting his own hope until he's able to sustain himself."

To show that hope has profound immunological effects, Barbara Peavey and her fellow psychologists at North Texas State University administered biofeedback training sessions in which participants learned to raise the temperature of their hands. Not surprisingly, psychological tests showed that individuals felt less stress than they had before. But blood tests showed that specific immune cells, phagocytes, were more potent after biofeedback.

And at Ohio State University, Janice Kiecolt-Glaser has found similar shifts in immune powers in geriatric patients after teaching them some standard relaxation exercises such as progressive relaxation (in which a person mentally travels through the body, selectively relaxing each part). Altered biochemical phenomena—presence of more active natural killer cells, for example—in the blood of the patients followed in the wake of doing relaxation exercises.

Harvard University psychologist David McClelland has been trying to find the key to self-healing through extensive thought and some experimentation. "It may turn out to be something fairly existential or religious," he has suggested. "A kind of personal disengagement combined with a kind of faith in something beyond the self, something beyond, or bigger than the self that you can trust."

Medically (as well as theologically), faith is an appropriate and potent companion to hope in the pharmacopia of PNI. Even traditional medicine pays some grudging deference to it in the form of a scientific anomaly known simply as placebo, a Latin word that means literally "I will please." A *placebo* is a medically inert substance or medical procedure with no known intrinsic therapeutic value that, nevertheless, is effective.

Placebos take many forms: colored pills, sham operations, or injections of harmless saltwater. For all their inert qualities, they have been used successfully to treat diseases from cancer to asthma to warts. For decades the placebo effect has been in some ways a nuisance in medicine. To prove that their products are not medically inert, pharmaceutical companies routinely test their latest products against placebos: pills or liquids that have the outward appearance of the real thing. In part through the necessity of dealing with the sometimes frustrating interference of the placebo effect, researchers inadvertently learned that the power of a new medicine, or a novel surgical procedure or therapy, is not always a simple matter of good chemistry, surgical skill, or "good" science.

To underscore the omnipresence of placebo power, placebo specialist Dr. David Sobel of Kaiser Hospital in California likes to point out that fads in medicines and treatments have always existed. Some of the weird and ghastly medicines of the past—crocodile dung, swine teeth, asses' hooves, frog sperm, eunuch fat, lozenges made from dried viper flesh, moss scraped from the skull of someone who died violently—worked as well as some of the Food and Drug Administration (FDA)-approved nostrums of the present.

Even today there are popular superstitions, or expectations, of certain medical paraphernalia. According to Dr. Sobel, injections are assumed to be more potent than pills, but pills themselves are very popular forms of medication (the average person, by one estimate, consumes 76,000 in a lifetime). One part of the pill's effectiveness is its appearance, particularly its size and color. In one study, researchers designed a poll to analyze the suggestive value of pill color and design. First, capsules, regardless of size, are considered more potent than tablets. Yellow or orange capsules, people think, are mood manipulators: stimulants or depressants; lavender pills are probably hallucinogens. Anything gray or dark red is judged to be a sedative. White pills, perhaps because of the aspirin imagery, are assumed to be painkillers and black pills are assumed to be hallucinogens.

One reason for the effectiveness of many placebos is unrelated to shape, color, and size. As Dr. Sobel points out, most diseases are *self-limiting;* that is, they run their course and end. At times, as Mark Twain put it, "God cures and the doctor sends the bill."

Another reason for their effectiveness is more personal: the efficacy of the placebo depends on belief in the treatment—old-fashioned faith. That belief must be shared by doctor and patient. Placebo expert Sobel likes to quote a nineteenth-century French doctor who said, "You should treat as many patients as possible with the new drugs while they still have the power to heal." The message is that doctors, just like everyone else, follow fads in medicine with the same waxing and waning of enthusiasm for a new medicine or therapy characteristic of the rest of humanity.

Belief is potent medicine. Doctors Herbert Benson of Harvard Medical School and David P. McCallie, Jr., of Harvard's Thorndike Laboratory were comparing various treatments for angina pectoris (heart pain). They found that an unusually high number of patients (approximately eight out of ten) reported relief from heart pain when treated by certain doctors. These highly successful doctors Benson and McCallie classified as "enthusiasts," because in each case the individual had introduced the therapy into medical practice. Naturally, they believed in their own work, and in some way they transmitted their faith and confidence to their patients. The effect was more than general good feelings of well-being: measurable improvements resulted. The enthusiasts' patients tolerated more strenuous exercise, reduced their nitroglycerin intake, and had improved electrocardiographic results. These improvements occurred even though, in some instances, the treatment was later shown to be ineffective.

Ritual adds to the strength of the patient's belief: visiting the doctor in the inner sanctum of the examining room or committing oneself to the temple of the hospital. Healers in other cultures have known this for centuries. Benson has gone so far as to suggest that much of the power of the placebo is due to simple caring. Every good doctor has something of the shaman, a talent for infecting people with hope and positive attitudes that heals as it uplifts.

Washington physician Dr. Morgan Martin wrote in the *Journal of the American Medical Association* about the knowledge of the healing ritual he gained from conversations with a Native American healer named Russell. Among the points Russell emphasized was that healer and patient share a belief about the nature of the world and disease; that the healer focus on not the disease but the reactions of family and friends to the disease; that the shaman involve a rich lore of ceremony in healing, in which others—the patient's family, the healer's helper—participate; that in the end the healer dispenses "a remedy and a ritual."

Most important, according to Russell, is faith in the healer. A medicine man consults with his support group of helpers, who interview a patient first. "He must believe in the medicine man," says Russell. "If the helpers say the patient does not believe, I may send him to a white doctor."

Once ignored in favor of Western medicine, traditional healing is today receiving more recognition. The National Institute of Mental Health has recognized this phenomenon for years and has had a program in New Mexico where apprentice Navajo medicine men learn the traditional ways of healing with ceremony, dances, rituals, and prayers.

The program was begun under the umbrella of the Minority Group Mental Health Program at NIMH to train tribespeople in the healing ways of the Navajo. It was initiated to fulfill a real medical and social need among them. While the Native Americans still revered and, for the most part, preferred the healing rituals of their ancestors, there were not many individuals continuing the medicine-man tradition. One reason was the difficulty of the undertaking. Many Navajo ceremonies are extremely elaborate. They require reciting long ceremonial prayers from memory. To perform one of the ceremonies it can take months, even years, of training. With funding from the NIMH program, forty people were trained in some of the healing rites of their people. Because of the effectiveness of Navajo medicine among its people, the NIMH found itself in the unusual position of preserving part of a cultural heritage for scientific reasons. (The healers often had better success than clinic doctors.) Programs are now starting elsewhere in the country—the Pacific Northwest, for example—to incorporate the best of the world of the shaman and the M.D. into a more effective healing system.

As a bizarre illustration of the real power of healer belief, David Sobel discusses a doctor treating an asthma patient who was having a particularly difficult time keeping his bronchial tubes open. As it happened the doctor had just heard about a potent new medicine and called the firm to ask for a sample. He gave it to the man. Improvement was spectacular; the patient was breathing more eas-ily in minutes, and his airways stayed clear for a longer time.

Curious about the real effect of the drug, the doctor decided to try an impromptu experiment and switched medication to an inert placebo to observe the result. The patient complained that some-thing was wrong with his latest prescription. He had some trouble breathing. Once he heard this, the doctor was convinced that he had found an effective new drug. He wrote to the pharmaceutical com-pany for more samples of the drug. A short time later, he was informed that he had received a placebo accidentally. Apparently it was *his* belief that the first was the genuine article that had helped his patient.

Healing of almost every sort demands belief. In a fascinating book, *Persuasion and Healing,* Dr. Jerome Frank, professor emeritus of psychiatry at the Johns Hopkins University, gives the dramatic example of an experiment done by a German doctor, whose subjects were three women ill enough to be bedridden. One was dying of cancer of the uterus that had spread throughout her body. A second had an inflamed gallbladder and chronic gallstones. The third was having difficulty recovering from abdominal surgery for an inflamed pancreas; over the seven months since the operation she had lost an excessive amount of weight and at the time of the experiment was skeletal.

Since conventional medicine had done all that was possible, the doctor decided to try faith healing. In the first part of the experiment, he asked a local healer who claimed to be able to heal without touching or even being nearby to help his three patients. On twelve different occasions, the healer tried to project his healing powers at the three patients. Nothing happened.

Then the doctor told the patients about the healer—about his amazing gift, his successes, the benefits of this healing technique, and so forth—and said that on a certain day the healer would be beaming his healing force at them; in fact, on that day the healer did nothing.

The day of the healing came and went. In the days that followed the woman who had been wasting away after her pancreas operation began to recover and gained thirty pounds. The patient with the gallstones lost all her symptoms and went home totally recovered. It was years before she had any more gallbladder problems. Although the cancer patient's disease had advanced to a lethal stage, the symptoms that had made her remaining weeks of life miserable receded. Her body, formerly puffy and bloated, excreted the excess fluids. Her strength returned; even her blood count improved slightly. She felt well enough to return home, where she lived the last three months of her life almost free of her debilitating symptoms.

Faith made these women physically stronger, in one instance strong enough to recover completely. Faith in the unseen, unfelt medical force was responsible for the dramatic transformation, but it would be a mistake to assume that only the belief in medical or quasi-medical rituals can work such marvels.

Frank also had a fascination with another manifestation of faith, so-called miracle cures: sudden and dramatic reversals of disease experienced by people who made a pilgrimage to Lourdes near the French Pyrenees. Legend has it that the Virgin Mary appeared here in 1858 to a French peasant girl, Bernadette Soubirous. Water from a spring discovered at the time of the apparition is believed to effect miraculous cures. Every year an estimated three million people, a half million of them sick people seeking a cure, travel to the shrine to drink and bathe in its icy waters. Since 1858, the Catholic

Church claims to have authenticated more than sixty instances of miracle cures that have occurred here. The ritual of making the pilgrimage, attending the ceremonies, praying at the shrine all played a part in this process of nonmedical healing, as Frank called it. So important is the ritual, he points out, that it had to be more than coincidence that, except for the very early days after the apparition appeared, no one from the Lourdes area experienced a cure.

Placebo expert David Sobel has suggested using this curative power by prescribing placebos to individuals and doing so ethically. One of the longstanding criticisms of using placebos in medicine is that the doctor deceives the patient by representing a sugar pill as effective. Sobel has suggested as an alternative a *double-blind situation*, in which neither the patient nor doctor knows whether a prescribed drug is placebo or actual medication. Another possibility is for the doctor to prescribe a placebo and to state that although the substance has no known chemical activity, it may relieve symptoms as hypnosis, biofeedback, and relaxation therapy do. With this sort of prelude the placebo—in whatever form it takes: a pill, a liquid, a simple exercise—can then be prescribed. Sobel firmly believes that placebos are effective, that they can be ethically administered to summon the placebo response, and that ultimately "the placebo makes a statement that we have within us a certain self-regulatory mechanism, a self-healing mechanism, which can be mobilized given proper situational and environmental cues."

The placebo response might also be mobilized by trying the relaxation response. In his years of observing individuals practice his exercises, Dr. Herbert Benson is convinced that the placebo response is the relaxation response. He has even begun to recommend to those who try his method that the key word they use to induce the response be a religious one, if that will be effective for them.

THERAPEUTIC TOUCH

Other nontraditional therapies may enter the mainstream of medicine in the near future. One that has been waiting in the wings for a long time is therapeutic or healing touch. The pioneer of this method is Dolores Krieger, a professor of nursing at New York

University and author of a book on the subject. After watching psychic healer Oskar Estebany in action, Krieger was convinced that relieving people's pain and distress by moving one's hands over them is a skill that can be learned. Since the mid-1970s she has conducted a course in therapeutic touch to thousands of people. Today more than fifty universities offer formal instruction in therapeutic touch, usually as part of the curriculum for nurses' training.

The ritual of therapeutic touch is reasonably simple. The healer first centers himself or herself. The healer eases into an altered state of consciousness as he concentrates or focuses his energies on the healing process at hand. The next step is to pass one's hands slowly over the person to be healed, four to six inches above the body of the patient, trying to sense energy beaming off the patient's body.

Krieger has been using the method for over a decade herself and says at the very least it produces a relaxation response in those treated and works well for fevers, inflammation, musculoskeletal problems, and psychosomatic diseases.

Still considered a medical oddity, therapeutic touch has only recently been receiving serious funding. In 1985, the first federal grant to study the phenomenon was awarded to Dr. Janet Quinn, of the University of South Carolina. In one experiment she conducted, two groups of healers passed their hands over two groups of heart patients in a New York City hospital. One group of healers had not centered themselves but were merely counting backward from 100 as they moved their hands in a ritualistic way over the patients. The other group was performing true healing: they had centered themselves and were concentrating on the person before them. The experiment was videotaped; no one watching could tell who was faking it and who was doing the real thing.

But the patients knew. The "healed" group showed a detectable drop in anxiety that the sham healers did not produce in their patients. The explanation by the healers is that some energy passed between them and their patients, but their interpretation has not been confirmed by proof. Some believe that this healing has no more than a placebo effect on those who receive it. That explanation is quite acceptable to Krieger and her fellow touchers, since it indicates that they have found a dependable way to summon that elusive response.

In the past few years more and more doctors and psychologists have been experimenting with another exercise, giving medical direction to a patient who is hovering between consciousness and unconsciousness. Accidental discoveries that some patients listen in to their own operations while they are under anesthesia suggest that the doctor can use or abuse that state of mind. Since the early 1960s one San Francisco physician, Dr. David Cheek, has claimed not only that anesthetized patients can hear what is said during an operation, but that what they hear may affect the outcome of the operation. To his colleagues' amusement, Cheek at one time proposed hanging a sign in the operating room cautioning: "Be Careful, The Patient is Listening."

For years Cheek's suggestion was at best treated as that of a well-meaning eccentric. Yet in his book on hypnotism, Canadian psychologist Kenneth Bowers cites an example in which a surgeon found a lump in a patient's mouth during some plastic surgery. The surgeon commented, "Good Gracious! It may not be a cyst at all. It may be cancer" and went on to finish the surgery. After the operation the patient was listless, depressed, and unaccountably tearful. Finally, under hypnosis, she was asked whether something was bothering her. Shortly afterward she blurted out: "Good Gracious! he is saying this is malignant!" Her depression lifted when she was reassured that the surgeon's snap diagnosis may not have been correct.

Other researchers have confirmed this item of medical folklore. Henry Bennett, a psychologist at the University of California Medical School at Davis, has been making systematic studies of the phenomenon. In one experiment, during operations he played a taped message that gave the suggestion that after the operation the patient would tug at an earlobe. Although none of the eleven patients remembered hearing the suggestion, nine did touch their lobes during a postoperation interview as requested.

Bennett believes that some patients hear the events that occur during surgery and that what they hear may affect postsurgical recovery. During a bone graft operation, one surgeon blurted out, "This is a terrible bone graft." Later the patient recalled having heard some negative comments about her graft. (As it happened, the graft was not effective, but whether failure resulted from the doctor acknowledging a medical fact or from his comment affecting the patient's response to the surgery is impossible to say.) At the very least, suggests Bennett, those who huddle around the patient in the operating theater should exercise some restraint.

As the preceding illustrate, scientific scrutiny is now applied to a recurrent theme of the lore of medicine: that some anesthetized patients hear and recall conversations that occur in the operating room. Now that he has found evidence of recall, Bennett plans to administer blood tests to surgical patients:

> We're looking at the level of stress hormones—epinephrine, norepinephrine, vasopressin—to see whether the degrees of stress that they're under correlates with their degree of memory. We suspect it will. When you go under anesthesia you're generally in a very highly stressed situation and you would be releasing a lot of these hormones. And there is evidence that these hormones have something to do with consolidating memories.

Bennett is going beyond observing to trying preoperative suggestion. On the day before an operation he sits with a patient and makes a series of suggestions. To a woman undergoing abdominal surgery he suggests that she try to shunt blood away from her abdomen and, after waking from surgery, keep her muscles flaccid to minimize the discomfort of recovery. Some surgeons, Bennett says, have commented on the small amount of bleeding in some of his prepared patients. "It gives them a sense of participation, a sense of continuity. It's a win-win situation," Bennett says, characterizing this method.

Pennsylvania State University hypnotherapist Howard Hall, who has reported inducing immune cell changes in people he has hypnotized, is planning to extend the use of the technique. Soon he hopes to study a group of cancer patients, using hypnosis to try to influence their immune systems. "If you look at the concept of disease as being some imbalance of a system—of the immune system being underreactive or overreactive—the question is: can psychological events regulate that? Can you give a specific suggestion: 'Slow down' or 'Speed up'?"

From Hall's perspective, his hypnosis experiments are returning us to an elemental form of medicine. "You know, the psychology of healing kept the human race alive long before the advent of modern medicine, a relatively recent development. But we've gotten lazy," he continues. "Our technology is so seductive. Let the pill do it, we think. But the pill can't always do it."

Hypnotism is only one of many options. PNI pioneer Robert Ader predicts the day when it will be possible to do with people what he did with his rats: condition the immune system by using certain cues. "When you administer drugs," explains Ader, "you are using a conditioning paradigm. Since there is a conditioning process going on, Ader points out, "Your only options are to study it or ignore it. It is there, so why ignore it?"

It already happens that some chemotherapy patients are negatively conditioned by their treatments. Most oncologists and nurses who treat cancer patients with chemotherapy are well aware of the phenomenon. Among the side effects of potent anticancer drugs is violent and excruciating nausea and patients being treated with these drugs can suffer from a conditioned reflex called anticipatory nausea and vomiting (ANV). One nurse who works in a cancer treatment clinic says that some patients describe feeling nauseated when they see the hospital or even begin to feel ill as they drive past the city limits where the hospital or clinic is located. For others the smell of the alcohol pads used to swab the skin in preparation for intravenous injections triggers nausea. Almost anything associated with the treatment may set off the attacks. As one oncologist was shopping in a supermarket, he rounded the corner and came face to face with one of his patients. Her first reaction on seeing him was to vomit.

Since a conditioning process occurs anyway, Robert Ader suggests that doctors use it in a positive way. For example, at some oncology clinic in the future a chemotherapy patient would undergo a special conditioning program in which diminishing doses of a cancer-fighting drug would be given along with increasing amounts of some harmless substance, a candy mint, for example. If Ader's thesis is correct, over time the patient's system would associate the flavor with the effects of the drug. The doctor could eventually reduce the chemotherapy dose and supplement it with the mints. In this way a physician could get the same medical results while using smaller doses of the drug.

TESTING

Because of the broader perspective PNI adds to disease, the process of gathering patient information will become more thorough than it already is. Besides taking a standard medical history, the conscientious doctor will need information about patients' psychological history: their current state of mind, moods, recent life crises, hardiness quotient, and dominant personality traits, among other variables.

In this instance, computerized information collection is especially valuable for managing a mass of data in a logical way. Psychoneuroimmunology entails integrating more data than various physiological specialties do, but not too many to be managed by a machine. It is possible now to program a desktop computer to generate a PNI profile of a patient. The computer would use for comparison a database of PNI variables and their influence on health. In the future such a system would be based on enough real case studies to generate useful and valuable probability predictions. The program would match family medical history, the individual's own medical history, a genetic fingerprint, and a psychological profile against what it has on file. It could then produce an estimate of a person's health and single out unhealthy elements of the PNI profile. The final decisions and prognosis would always be made by a flesh-and-blood analyst, but that physician would have a more sophisticated base of information upon which to draw conclusions.

Already computer programs can generate medical diagnoses. The University of Pittsburgh has developed a so-called expert system for a large computer called *Caduceus* that can diagnose more than six hundred medical diseases. Doctors who have access to a personal computer already have the option of using scaled-down versions of expert systems in their practice. (A diagnostic system called *Puff* has been developed by a lung specialist for his patients. The program, stored on a computer disk, makes a diagnosis based on the information the doctor feeds into the computer.)

The time may come when a patient can speak for five minutes into a microphone connected to a computer, the doctor can run the speech analysis program, and a print-out indicating the type and intensity of emotional distress the person is experiencing will be produced. The computer could analyze the synergy of various elements of behavioral medicine, including physiological measures of stress, and by mixing and matching different factors give a doctor access to risk factor equations of sickness and health. The program might show that when certain combinations of factors (diet, personality, genetics, smoking habits) are taken into consideration, a person stood 5 percent increase in the risk of developing cancer in his or her lifetime. Clues about the types of cancer the person would be most likely to develop would then indicate appropriate diagnostic tests. Similarly, recommendations for risk-factor reduction could be made.

Since depression is a strong psychological element in disease susceptibility, simple precautionary tests for depression may also be possible. No less prestigious an organization than the National Academy of Science's Institute of Medicine, in a report studying the effects of stress on illness, suggested that medical research should enlist some of the new technologies to help analyze the contributions of this tricky and complex factor.

The study recommended that researchers place greater emphasis on gene mapping since all the major biochemical components of stress reactions are ultimately under genetic control and people have permanent, heritable differences in their reaction to stress. This is particularly important since some researchers have already identified (in individual mice and rats) genes that control the ways hormones are made and are moved to other parts of the body and even the reactions of individual organs. These researchers are on the verge of constructing a gene map for humans, as well, charting individuals' inherited style of responding to stress.

The genetic factor in stress, according to the Institute's panel, has practically been ignored. The way genetic differences are influenced by psychological factors—upbringing, life experiences, feelings of self-esteem or inadequacy—is not known. Nor is the question of the effect of personality and behavior on the genes. Through an understanding about the interaction of these elements, the panel predicts, physicians would gain access to a list of biochemical markers "to identify people who are at particular risk following stressful life events."

"NATURAL DRUGS"

Since anything that enters the body, including medication, can potentially shape the functioning of the immune system for better or worse, the hidden influences of the material we ingest is receiving increasing attention. Some researchers are worried about the effect of nutrition on brain chemistry and on the immune system itself. After a decade of work in this area, Richard Wurtman of the Massachusetts Institute of Technology has begun to isolate nutrients that affect the functioning of the brain and the nervous system. Among the findings he and his colleagues have made is that the amino acid tyrosine is an important food component since it forms the raw material for, among other substances, norepinephrine. High-protein meals are the primary source of this substance, which, says psychiatrist Alan Gelenberg of Harvard Medical School, also acts as a mild antidepressant.

In a very young and controversial field of research, neurophysiologist David Horrobin of the Clinical Research Institute in Montreal maintains that a certain hormonelike substance called *prostaglandin E_1* is a nutritional commodity that is tremendously important to a smoothly functioning immune system. This Oxford University–educated scientist has also claimed that through diet a person could manipulate the immune system, particularly the cancer-fighting T-cells.

We know there are large deposits of prostaglandin E_1 in the thymus, where the immune system's T-cells mature. Mice specifically bred to develop defective T-cells and overactive B-cells eventually succumb to the mouse equivalent of the autoimmune disease lupus erythematosus. Horrobin has found that when these animals are given prostaglandin E_1, their T-cells regain their normal function, the B-cells are under normal control, and the animals live longer.

The primary sources of the raw material for prostaglandin E_1, says Horrobin, are essential fatty acids found largely in vegetable oils. But to use the raw material fully, the body also needs adequate supplies of other nutrients: zinc, vitamin B_6, and vitamin C. Horrobin is grappling with the problem of the amounts of these nutrients we need each day. At the moment his findings suggest that the body requires 20 to 25 milligrams of vitamin B_6, 5 to 15 milligrams of zinc, 250 to 500 milligrams of vitamin C, and a special kind of vegetable oil, primrose oil, which is particularly rich in the kinds of essential fatty acids that are easily transformed into prostaglandin E_1. "By careful attention to diet," he declares, "it should be possible to activate T-lymphocyte function in a large number of diseases, including rheumatoid arthritis, various autoimmune diseases, multiple sclerosis, and cancer, in which [immune] function is defective."

For reasons that are still not clarified, simple foods such as milk, two to three glasses per day, decrease a person's risk of developing colorectal cancer. Epidemiologist Richard Shekelle and his coresearchers compared the health with the dietary histories of more than nineteen hundred men whose medical status was monitored for eleven years. The observers noted that men who developed colorectal cancer also had lower vitamin D intake, either because of their diet or because they lived in a low-sunlight area. As an antidote to the vitamin deficiency, one doctor has recommended two or three glasses of nonfat, vitamin D–enriched milk per day.

On the basis of current knowledge about some of the subtle mechanisms of the immune system, other researchers have been trying to exploit natural mechanisms to enhance the body's immune strength. For example, the discovery that white blood cells have receptors for the brain's natural opiates, enkephalins, and seem to become more potent through the interaction has prompted Nicholas Plotnikoff, professor of pharmacology at Oral Roberts University, to use injections of enkephalins to enhance the cancer-fighting ability of the body.

Plotnikoff tested the injections on a group of leukemia-stricken mice. A first group received injections; a second group received none. By the end of two weeks the second group was dead; the enkephalin group lived four weeks. In another experiment he took blood samples from a group of cancer patients who had Hodgkin's disease and poured some enkephalins into the blood sample. A noticeable surge in the immunopotency of the cancer victims' white blood cells resulted.

These results prompted Plotnikoff to take the next step: injecting the enkephalin directly into the cancer patient. In fall 1983 he received permission from the Food and Drug Administration to launch the first approved use of brain opiates on cancer patients. His strategy is to determine whether enkephalin injections help to stimulate the tumor-killing abilities of the immune system. Plotnikoff theorizes that chronic stress depletes the body's quota of enkephalins; part of his experimental approach he calls *enkephalin replacement therapy,* using synthetic enkephalin. As an anticancer therapy, his procedure is still highly experimental and expensive. When Plotnikoff began his work on humans in 1983, synthetic enkephalin cost $1,000 a gram, but since it now costs one-fifth that amount, Plotnikoff expects the price to continue to fall.

TENDER LOVING CARE

If what we have already learned about health and healing is accurate, the healing institutions, specifically the hospitals of this country, should start making some major transformations. One such change can be done with the help of a Colorado-based consulting firm that specializes in "patient relations," basically the business of teaching hospitals to be more hospitable. They give hospital staffs seminars on human relations, communications, even a "niceness training program." As a result of its advice, some hospitals have not only revamped their manners but their look as well. One hospital in Colorado has carpeted hallways, a uniformed doorman (an unpaid volunteer), new mattresses and linens, carnations on every dinner tray. The reason for the popularity of the consulting firm is purely financial—hospitals are competing more and more for the health care dollar. The effects may be more profound. Consider these three hospital vignettes.

The first centers around an eight-year obsession of Roger Ulrich, a researcher with the geography department of the University of Delaware. Over that time he asked the nurses on one floor of a Pennsylvania hospital to keep notes on patients who came in for gallbladder operations and were randomly assigned rooms. He asked them to document the amount of painkillers and antianxiety medication each patient used after surgery, postsurgical minor complications, and the length of their hospital stay.

At the end of the eight-year span, Ulrich gathered up all the data and analyzed them. One group typically took more painkillers, had slightly more postoperative complaints, and generally stayed in the hospital longer to recover from the surgery. Since their chief common denominator was the miserable view from their room (a bland, featureless brick wall), he called them the "wall-view patients."

Another group used fewer painkillers, were rated by the nurses as having fewer complaints, and on the average went home from the hospital about a day and a half sooner than the wall-view group. Ulrich called the healthier crowd the "tree-view group" because their windows looked out on a small stand of trees. Since the view actually seemed to affect the quality of health of the patients studied, Ulrich mused that the people who design hospitals should pay more attention to the location of buildings and intangibles such as "the quality of patient window views."

In another situation, psychologist Ellen Langer selected a random group of surgical patients (gallbladder, hysterectomy, hernia repair) at Yale–New Haven Hospital in New Haven, and tried to work some fundamental changes in their inner and outer experience of recovering from surgery. She divided them into groups and prepared each for postoperative recovery in a slightly different way.

She asked one group some simple questions about what they expected to happen to them while they were patients. She gave a second group basic information about the surgery: surgical preparation, the reasons for those procedures, the aftereffects of surgery, and probable minor pain and discomfort that would occur.

Langer gave a third group what she called a *coping device,* basically a brief primer on techniques to deal with the physical discomfort of surgery. For example, she explained that pain and discomfort are relative; she pointed out that although people seldom noticed receiving a minor cut while playing football or hurrying to finish preparation for an elaborate party, people who suffered small paper cuts while reading a boring book were more than likely to lavish attention on the hurt. Her point was that people have more of their body under their control than they may realize. Langer also took the time to emphasize positive aspects of being in the hospital. First, the person would eventually feel better. The hospital stay would give them an excuse to pamper themselves a little: to relax, luxuriate in being cared for, maybe even to lose a few pounds, if they wanted to reduce their weight. She taught them to emphasize the bright side of the experience.

After surgery she compared the groups, paying special attention to their recovery, use of pain relievers and sedatives, and duration of hospital stay. The first and second group were not noticeably different in the number of days they needed to recover from the surgery and the amount of medication they took. However, the third group, those who had had the short coping primer, used half as many painkillers and sedatives and stayed in the hospital an average of two days less than the second group.

The difference in recovery, suggests Langer, was due to the patients' learning that they could diminish postsurgical discomfort and in so doing feel that they were in control. Perhaps such a coping device could be incorporated in the patients' initial interview when they enter the hospital.

The third illustration is related to David McClelland's fascination with the phenomenon of healing revolving around what he calls the *Mother Teresa effect* (Mother Teresa is the Nobel Laureate who has dedicated her life to the poor of Calcutta). McClelland was intrigued that after a group of students watched a gritty, emotionally involving documentary, blood tests indicated that their immune systems had slightly higher levels of an immunoglobulin. The effect was temporary (it only lasted an hour), but it was real.

He later worked on a variation of the Mother Teresa effect. Instead of showing them the film, he asked his graduate students to spend an hour thinking deeply about two subjects: a time in their life when they felt that someone loved and cared for them and a time when they loved somebody. He had already tried the technique on himself and believed that it is effective. "Now when I'm getting a cold I spend some time thinking about loving relationships. A couple of times it even stopped my cold. It isn't foolproof," he admits. "Once I got terribly sick in spite of it all. But it helps."

McClelland's belief in the power of love has marked the direction he advocates for modern medicine. It should use the overlooked resources of the mind and human spirit, which are, McClelland is convinced, the source of the inner forces of healing. "I can dream a little about changing hospital environments," he once told a gathering of his colleagues, "one that relaxes you, gives you loving care, and relieves you of the incessant desire to control and run everything. A healthful environment. Certain doctors, nurses, social workers—all of us—can learn, it seems to me, that being loving to people is really good for their health. And probably good for yours too."

Appendixes

Stress Measurement

THE HOLMES-RAHE
SOCIAL READJUSTMENT RATING SCALE

Some events in life surprise us pleasantly, some not. Although it is hardly a definitive list, the Holmes-Rahe Social Readjustment Rating Scale will give some idea of what those events might be and how significant they are in their psychological impact on us:

Event	Number value
Death of a spouse	100
Divorce	73
Marital separation	65
Jail term	63

Death of close family member 63
Personal injury or illness 53
Marriage 50
Fired from work 47
Marital reconciliations 45
Retirement 45
Change in family member's health 44
Pregnancy 40
Sex difficulties 39
Addition to family 39
Business readjustment 39
Change in financial status 38
Death of close friend 37
Change to different line of work 36
Change in number of marital arguments 35
Mortgage or loan over $10,000 31
Foreclosure of mortgage or loan 30
Change in work responsibilities 29
Son or daughter leaving home 29
Trouble with in-laws 29
Outstanding personal achievement 28
Spouse begins or stops work 26
Starting or finishing school 26
Change in living conditions 25
Revision of personal habits 24
Trouble with boss 23
Change in work hours, conditions 20
Change in residence 20
Change in schools 20
Change in recreational habits 19
Change in church activities 19
Change in social activities 18
Mortgage or loan under $10,000 17
Change in sleeping habits 16
Change in number of family gatherings 15
Change in eating habits 15
Vacation 13
Christmas season 12
Minor violation of the law 11

In theory, any score over 300 in a year's time, according to Holmes and Rahe, would suggest a person had a high probability (80 percent chance) of becoming seriously ill.

POSSIBLE INDICATORS OF EXCESSIVE STRESS

1. Physical symptoms and conditions:

    headaches
    high blood pressure
    palpitations
    disturbed sleep
    loss of appetite
    dry mouth
    peptic ulcers
    chest pain
    diarrhea
    grinding teeth
    hyperventilation
    backache
    asthma
    skin rashes
    excessive sweating
    hives

2. Psychological symptoms:

    Disturbed moods
        depression
        anger
        inappropriate and excessive elation
        rapid, dramatic mood changes
        anxiety

    Disturbances of thinking

        impaired attention
        impaired concentration

impaired memory
confusion
irrational fears
indecisiveness
self-consciousness
disorganization
ideas of injuring oneself or another

Disturbances of behavior

changes in appearance: sloppy dress, poor self-care
abnormal movements: restlessness, pacing, fidgeting,
  nailbiting
abnormal speech: stuttering, halting, stammering
habits: drug abuse, alcohol abuse, excessive coffee or
  tea consumption, overeating, binge eating, starting,
  resuming, or increasing cigarette smoking
sexual problems: loss of interest in sex, impotence,
  loss of orgasmic ability, sexual promiscuity
impaired performance at work
phobias

3. Family and social problems:

marital problems
children's school or behavior problems

Books and Periodicals

BOOKS

Achterberg, Jeanne. *Imagery in Healing: Shamanism and Modern Medicine.* San Francisco: Shambhala Publications, 1985. A succinct and often poetic description of the use of imagery throughout the history of medicine, from the days of the shaman to the present.

Ader, Robert. *Psychoneuroimmunology.* New York: Academic Press, 1981. A highly technical yet seminal text on the field.

Alexander, Franz, M.D. *Psychosomatic Medicine.* New York: W. W. Norton, 1950. An almost prescient work by the man responsible for the existence of psychosomatic medicine in this country.

Benson, Herbert, with Miriam Z. Klipper. *The Relaxation Response.* New York: Avon, 1976. A mandatory purchase for anyone seriously interested in using the mind to keep the body well. The originator of the Relaxation Response explains it clearly and succinctly.

Cousins, Norman. *Anatomy of an Illness.* New York: Bantam Books, 1981. The book that popularized many of the notions of psychoneuroimmunology before it had a name.

Ellenberger, Henri F. *The Discovery of the Unconscious.* New York: Basic Books, 1970. The seeds of what became the core features of PNI are discussed in this readable history of psychiatry.

Frank, Jerome D. *Persuasion and Healing.* New York: Schocken Books: 1974. Arguably the best popularity written book on the subject of healing. It's a fascinating study of medicine's flirtation with the essence of psychoneuroimmology for centuries.

Pelletier, Kenneth R. *Mind as Healer, Mind as Slayer.* New York: Dell Publishing Co., 1977. A book that has become a modern classic on the subject of holistic medicine. It takes a sane, balanced approach to presenting and describing the often confusing and sometimes contradictory field of medicine.

Seyle, Hans. *The Stress of Life.* New York: McGraw-Hill, 1976. Written by the man who originated the concept, it is the most informative book on stress.

Simonton, O. Carl, M.D., Stephanie Matthews-Simonton, and James L. Creighton. *Getting Well Again.* New York: Bantam Books, 1981. A clear explanation of what has come to be known simply as the Simonton technique of using imagery to combat cancer.

Sontag, Susan. *Illness as Metaphor.* New York: Vintage Books, 1978. A quirky, stimulating discussion of the mythic stature of cancer from the viewpoint of a very articulate cancer patient.

Spingarn, Natalie Davis. *Hanging in There: Living Well on Borrowed Time.* New York: Stein and Day, 1983. Personal testament, this one written by a cancer patient for other cancer patients. Full of down-to-earth, practical advice.

Starr, Paul. *The Social Transformation of American Medicine.* New York: Basic Books, 1983. A fascinating study of how politics and not science determines the type of medicine practiced in America today.

POPULAR MAGAZINES

For general information that is solid and up-to-date and attuned to new developments in PNI, the monthly *American Health* magazine is worth the subscription price ($14.95 per year at this writing). For subscription information write:

American Health: Fitness of
Mind and Body
P.O. Box 10035
Des Moines, IA

or:
80 Fifth Avenue, Suite 302
New York, NY 10011

OTHER POPULAR MAGAZINES INCLUDE:

New Age Journal
342 Western Avenue
Brighton, MA 02135

Psychology Today
535 N. Dearborn Street
Chicago, IL 60610

Prevention
33 East Minor Street
Emmaus, PA 18049

FOR THE MORE TECHNICALLY ORIENTED:

America's Health
Worldwide Medical Press, Inc.
257 Park Avenue South
New York, NY 10010

Medical Tribune
641 Lexington Avenue
New York, NY 10022

Medical World News
1221 Avenue of the Americas
New York, NY 10020

Behavioral Medicine Abstracts
Society of Behavioral
Medicine
P.O. Box 8530
Knoxville, TN 37996

Behavioral Medicine Update
Society of Behavioral
Medicine
P.O. Box 8530
Knoxville, TN 37996

Brain/Mind Bulletin
P.O. Box 42211
Los Angeles, CA 90004

Executive Fitness Newsletter
Rodale Press, Inc.
33 East Minor Street
Emmaus, PA 18049

Harvard Medical School
Health Letter
79 Garden Street
Cambridge, MA 02138

Healthline
1320 Bayport Avenue
San Carlos, CA 94070

Inquiring Mind
P.O. Box 9999
North Berkeley Station
Berkeley, CA 94709

Newsletter of the AABM
The American Academy of
Behavioral Medicine
8616 Northwest Plaza Drive,
Suite 210
Dallas, TX 75225

JOURNALS

Advances
Available on a quarterly basis
by becoming a member of
The Institute for the
Advancement of Health
16 East 53rd Street
New York, NY 10022.
Members' annual fee is $35 at
this writing. The best and
most readable journal for the
clinician and sophisticated lay
reader on mind-body aspects
of health and disease.

American Journal of Clinical
Hypnosis
American Society of Clinical
Hypnosis
2250 East Devon Avenue,
Suite 336
Des Plaines, IL 60018

American Psychologist
American Psychological
Association
1200 17th Street, N.W.
Washington, DC 20036

Archives of Dermatology
American Medical Association
535 N. Dearborn Street
Chicago, IL 60610

Biofeedback and
Self-Regulation
Biofeedback Society of
America
4301 Owens Street
Wheat Ridge, CO 80033

British Journal of Holistic
Medicine
179 Gloucester Place
London NW1 6DX
England

Cancer
American Cancer Society
777 Third Avenue
New York, NY 10017

General Hospital Psychiatry
Elsevier Science Publishing
Company, Inc.
52 Vanderbilt Avenue
New York, NY 10017

Health Psychology
Lawrence Erlbaum
Association, Inc.
365 Broadway, Suite 102
Hillsdale, NJ 07642

Humane Medicine
399 Bathurst Street
Toronto, Ontario M5T 2S8
Canada

International Journal of
Clinical and Experimental
Hypnosis
Society for Clinical and
Experimental Hypnosis
129-A Kings Park Drive
Liverpool, NY 13088

Journal of the American
Medical Association
American Medical Association
535 N. Dearborn Street
Chicago, IL 60610

Journal of Behavioral
Medicine
Plenum Press
226 West 17th Street
New York, NY 10011

Journal of Complementary
Medicine
21 Portland Place
London W1N 3HF
England

Journal of Human Stress
Opinion Publications
Rural Route 1
Box 396
Shelburne Falls, MA 01370

New England Journal of
Medicine
10 Shattuck Street
Boston, MA 02115

Psychological Medicine
Cambridge University Press
32 East 57th Street
New York, NY 10022

Psychosomatic Medicine
American Psychosomatic
Society
265 Nassau Road
Roosevelt, NY 11575

Psychosomatics
American Academy of
Psychosomatic Medicine
70 West Hubbard Street, Suite
202
Chicago, IL 60610

Resources and Organizations

The following is a selection of therapeutic, research, and funding organizations dedicated to treating and curing a variety of diseases and medical conditions. The first group listed is for the lay public, the second for health care professionals. We have tried to select carefully each organization mentioned. But remember, in seeking out medical advice, your best ally in deciding what advice and guidance to follow is a doctor who knows you and your medical history and who has your trust and respect.

AIDS

National Gay Task Force
The only national source of information on current therapies and
research breakthroughs, it operates a toll-free hotline:
    800-221-7044
    Monday–Friday, 3:00 P.M.– 9:00 P.M. (EST)

Local groups include:

Gay Men's Health Crisis
    Box 274
    132 West Twenty-fourth Street
    New York, NY 10011
    212-685-4952
The GMHC sends crisis counselors to AIDS patients' homes, sponsors patients support in other ways: has a twenty-four-hour hotline,
provides a buddy system for those who need assistance in
housekeeping, and helps fund AIDS research.

People with AIDS
Support networks set up locally for those with AIDS. This is prolif-
erating all the time. Check local directory for information on any in
your area.

AIDS Medical Foundation
    230 Park Avenue
    Suite 1266
    New York, NY 10017
    212-949-7410
Raises funds for AIDS research.

Allergies

Allergy Foundation of America
    1302 18th Street, N.W.
    Suite 303
    Washington, DC 20036

National research organization dedicated to finding the cause and improving the therapies for treating allergies.

Arthritis

Arthritis Information Clearinghouse
P.O. Box 9782
Arlington, VA 22209
703-558-8250

As its name suggests, this is a clearinghouse of information for scientist and layman alike for new and updated information on arthritis and musculoskeletal diseases. It is sponsored by the National Institute of Arthritis, Diabetes, and Digestive and Kidney Diseases.

Stanford University Arthritis Center
HRP Building, Room 6
Stanford, CA 94305

Makes available relaxation tapes for arthritics.

Aids for Arthritis, Inc.
3 Little Knoll Court
Medford, NJ 08055

To make life a little easier, this organization has available inexpensive self-help tools for arthritics who have trouble performing some of the simple daily tasks of life—opening doors, manipulating switches.

Arthritis Foundation
1314 Spring Street N.W.
Atlanta, GA 30309
404-872-7100

Blood Diseases

National Association For Sickle Cell Disease
3460 Wilshire Blvd., Suite 1012
Los Angeles, CA 90010
213-731-1166

Provides both technical assistance—screening and testing possible carriers—and support services such as blood banks, summer camps for children with the disease, vocational rehabilitation.

National Hemophilia Foundation
  19 West Thirty-fourth Street
  Room 1204
  New York, NY 10001
  212-563-0211

An organization of volunteers, hemophiliacs and nonhemophiliacs, that supports research into the disease, operates referral services for patients and summer camps for children.

Cancer

Cancer patients or families of cancer patients who need more information about the disease or guidance on what to do can call either the American Cancer Society, in New York City, or the Cancer Information Service, an information number, offered by the National Cancer Institute, that can guide anyone interested to counseling centers. Each organization has several support programs available to patients and their families. For information on what there is, we provide the following addresses and phone numbers:

American Cancer Society
  777 Third Avenue
  New York, NY 10017
  212-371-2900

Among the programs the American Cancer Society offers are the following:

- *CanSurmount:* an educational and support program that includes recovered cancer patients as advisers and guides to educating patients and their families about the disease

- *I Can Cope:* a psychological support system for cancer patients

- International Association of Laryngectomees: support organization set up to help people who have had laryngectomies get back into the mainstream of life and employment

- Reach to Recovery: physical and psychological rehabilitation for women who have had mastectomies.

Local phone numbers for the Cancer Information Service administered by the National Cancer Institute:

Alaska	800-638-6070
California	
(from area codes 213,	
714, and 805)	800-252-9066
Colorado	800-332-1850
Connecticut	800-922-0824
Delaware	800-523-3586
District of Columbia	
(includes suburban Maryland	
and northern Virginia)	202-636-5700
Florida	800-432-5953
Georgia	800-327-7332
Hawaii	800-524-1234
Illinois	800-972-0586
Kentucky	800-432-9321
Maine	800-225-7034
Maryland	800-492-1444
Massachusetts	800-952-7420
Minnesota	800-582-5262
Montana	800-525-0231
New Hampshire	800-225-7034
New Jersey	800-523-3586
New Mexico	800-525-0231
New York City	212-794-7982
New York State	800-462-7255
North Carolina	800-672-0943
North Dakota	800-328-5188
Ohio	800-282-6522
Pennsylvania	800-822-3963
South Dakota	800-328-5188
Texas	800-392-2040
Vermont	800-225-7034
Washington	800-552-7212
Wisconsin	800-362-8038

Wyoming   800-525-0231
All other areas   800-638-6694

Other organizations:

Cancer Connection
    H&R Block Building
    4410 Main
    Kansas City, MO 64111
    816-932-8453
This matches cancer patients with others who have either been
cured or are in remission. The idea is to provide the newly diagnosed
patient with support from someone who has been through the
ordeals of the disease. It operates hotlines throughout parts of the
South and the East. Write or call to see if their services are available
in your area.

Children's Cancer Fund of America
    P.O. Box 374
    351 Plandome Road
    Manhasset, NY 11030
    516-627-6407
Raises funds for research into fighting cancer in children.

Committee for Freedom of Choice in Cancer Therapy
    111 Ellis Street, Suite 300
    San Francisco, CA 94102
    415-981-8384
Acts as an outlet for patients who want to become informed about
current cancer therapies and tries to educate the general public, but
does not interfere between an informed patient and his physician.

International Association of Cancer Victims and Friends
    7740 West Manchester Avenue, No. 110
    Playa Del Rey, CA 90291
Supports independent research on "nontoxic" therapies and cam-
paigns to clean carcinogens out of our food and water.

Leukemia Society of America
    733 Third Avenue
    New York, NY 10017
    212-573-8484

Acts as an information resource on the disease, supports research, and offers patient services, including aid to needy patients.

The Concern for Dying
  250 West Fifty-seventh Street
  New York, NY 10019
An organization that concerns itself with providing copies of the living will, which enables a patient to record his wishes concerning his treatment.

Make Today Count
  P.O. Box 303
  Burlington, IA 52601
There are more than two hundred chapters of this organization, which provides emotional support in dealing with the disease one day at a time.

The National Hospice Organization
  301 Tower, Suite 506
  301 Maple Avenue West
  Vienna, VA 22181
A referral service for terminally ill patients, made up of groups that provide hospice care or guidelines for taking care of the terminally ill.

United Cancer Council, Inc.
  1803 North Meridian Street
  Indianapolis, IN 46202
This is a federation of voluntary agencies, supported by the United Way, that fund cancer research and provide patient education and therapy groups.

United Ostomy Association
  1111 Wilshire Boulevard
  Los Angeles, CA 90017
An organization that provides moral support to patients who have had ostomies (such as a colostomy) and education on how to live with the operation's results.

Regional organizations and programs:

Cancer Call
PAC (People Against Cancer)
American Cancer Society
  37 South Wabash Avenue
  Chicago, IL 60603
This organization offers telephone support to cancer patients from recovered cancer patients.

Cancer Care, Inc. of the National Cancer Foundation
  One Park Avenue
  New York, NY 10016
A system of volunteers that provides professional counseling to cancer patients and their families.

TOUCH, Coordinator, Cancer Control Program
  University of Alabama
  104 Old Hillman Building
  Birmingham, AL 35294
A program whose goal is to instill in cancer patients and their families realistic and positive attitudes toward cancer treatment.

Psychosocial Counseling Service
  UCLA-Johnson Comprehensive Cancer Center
  1100 Glendon Avenue
  Suite 844
  Los Angeles, CA 90024
Professional mental-health counseling by phone for cancer patients, their families, and friends.

Diabetes Mellitus

American Diabetes Association
  2 Park Avenue
  New York, NY 10016
  212-683-7444
The national research organization for this disease. Funds diabetes research and disseminates information about the disease.

Juvenile Diabetes Foundation International
   60 Madison Avenue U
   New York, NY 10010
   212-889-7575
Seeks funds for research and provides support services to juvenile diabetics and their families.

Headache

National Migraine Foundation
   5252 Northwestern Avenue
   Chicago, IL 60625

Herpes

Herpes Resource Center
   P.O. Box 100
   Palo Alto, CA 94302
   415-328-7710 (8:00 A.M.–1:00 P.M.)
A national information source on the latest treatment and therapies and where they are given.

Lupus Erythematosus

The American Lupus Society
   23751 Madison Street
   Torrance, CA 90505
   213-373-1335
Disseminates information about the disease, supports research, and its local chapters hold meetings of lupus patients for mutual support.

Leanon (Lupus Erythematosus Anonymous)
   c/o Betty Hull
   P.O. Box 10243
   Corpus Christi, TX 78410

233

Lupus patients are invited to share their experiences and ways of coping with the disease with other lupus sufferers.

Lupus Foundation of America
    11921A Olive Boulevard
    St. Louis, MO 63141
    314-872-9036
A national nonprofit group that provides education, service, and emotional support for lupus sufferers.

Multiple Sclerosis

National Multiple Sclerosis Society
    205 East Forty-second Street
    New York, NY 10017

Skin Diseases

National Psoriasis Foundation
    6415 S.W. Canyon Court, Suite 200
    Portland, OR 97221
    503-297-1545
In addition to supporting research into the disease, this organization has group therapy and even a pen-pal program for teenage psoriasis sufferers.

International Scleroderma Federation
    135 Madison Avenue
    New York, NY 10016
    212-684-5023
Provides funds for research into scleroderma and support for sufferers of this disease.

United Scleroderma Foundation
    P.O. Box 350
    Watsonville, CA 95077
    408-728-2202
Coordinates information about the disease for the medical profession and the lay public. It operates a support network for scleroderma sufferers.

Miscellaneous

National Self-Help Clearing House
    33 West Forty-second Street
    New York, NY 10036
    212-840-7606

Alternative Medical Therapies

For medical topics that straddle what might be called the PNI-holistic boundaries, one of the most valuable sources of reliable information about new therapies and holistic health conferences is:

Interface
    230 Central Street
    Newton, MA 02166

Other valuable information and referral sources for alternative therapies include:

American Holistic Medical Association
    6932 Little River Turnpike
    Annandale, VA 22003
    703-642-5880
This will refer the public to certified physicians who are experienced in using nontraditional therapies such as acupuncture and behavioral medicine.

American Holistic Health Sciences Association
    1766 Cumberland Green, Suite 208
    St. Charles, IL 60174
    312-377-1929
This acts as an information resource for patients on holistic therapies that have some medical value.

BEHAVIOR AND PSYCHOSOMATIC MEDICINE SOCIETIES

These are largely designed for health care professionals, although they can be a valuable resource for patients seeking referrals.

Biofeedback Societies

Anyone interested in searching out clinics and-or physicians using biofeedback as part of medical therapy can write:

Biofeedback Society of America
  c/o Francine Butler, Ph.D.
  4301 Owens Street
  Wheat Ridge, CO 80033
  303-420-2889

American Association of Biofeedback Clinicians
  2424 Dempster
  Des Plaines, IL 60016
  312-827-0440

This group operates a national certification program for biofeedback practitioners and has a public registry of biofeedback practitioners.

Human Development

These are institutions that teach techniques commonly used in PNI—meditation, relaxation methods, imagery—and as part of their regimen provide training in using those methodologies.

Esalen Institute
  Big Sur, CA 93920
  408-667-2335

Institute for the Study of Human Knowledge
  Box 176
  Altos, CA 94022
  415-948-9428

Lama Foundation
  Box 444
  San Cristobal, NM 87564

Conducts seminars on meditation, yoga, music, ancient religious traditions. Offers communal life of self-realization.

Association for the Development of Human Potential
    Box 60
    Porthill, ID 83853
    604-227-9224

Interface
    230 Central Street
    Newton, MA 02166

Hypnosis

International Society For Professional Hypnosis
    218 Monroe Street
    Boonton, NJ 07005
    201-335-4334
Offers a referral service of health professionals who use hypnosis in their practice. It is also a professional society for counselors, doctors, nurses, psychologists, and others who use hypnotherapy.

National Society of Hypnotherapists
    P.O. Box 7586
    Newark, DE 19711
    302-737-8029
Professional society offering a referral service to professional hypnotists.

Meditation

Dharma Foundation
    P.O. Box 9999
    North Berkeley Station
    Berkeley, CA 94709

Psychotherapy

American Association for Marriage and Family Therapy
    1000 Connecticut Avenue, N.W., Suite 407
    Washington, DC 20036
A professional society of marriage and family therapists that operates a referral service as well.

American Psychological Association
    1200 17th Street, N.W.
    Washington, DC 20036
The professional organization for psychologists. Publishes various professional journals for psychologists.

American Psychiatric Association
    1400 K Street, N.W.
    Washington, DC 20004
The professional society for psychiatrists.

Psychoanalysis

Association for Advancement of Psychoanalysis
    329 East Sixty-second Street
    New York, NY 10021
    212-752-5267
Fosters training in psychoanalysis and offers a referral service.

National Psychological Association for Psychoanalysis
    150 West Thirteenth Street
    New York, NY 10011
    212-924-7440
A professional organization that offers a referral service and operates a library accessible to the public.

PROFESSIONAL AND SCIENTIFIC RESEARCH ORGANIZATIONS

AIDS

AIDS Medical Foundation
  230 Park Avenue
  Suite 1266
  New York, NY 10017
  212-949-7410
Raises funds for AIDS research.

Allergy

Allergy Foundation of America
  1302 18th Street N.W.
  Suite 303
  Washington, DC 20036

Arthritis

Arthritis Foundation
  1314 Spring Street N.W.
  Atlanta, GA 30309
  404-872-7100

Arthritis Information Clearinghouse
  P.O. Box 9782
  Arlington, VA 22209
  703-558-8250
As its name suggests, this is a clearinghouse of information on arthritis and musculoskeletal diseases. It is sponsored by the National Institute of Arthritis, Diabetes, and Digestive and Kidney Diseases.

Institute for Research of Rheumatic Diseases
  Box 955, Ansonia Station
  New York, NY 10023
  212-595-1368

Through its bimonthly newsletter, *Arthritis: Nutrition Stress News,* it disseminates the latest information on arthritis research.

Blood Diseases

National Association for Sickle Cell Disease
    3460 Wilshire Blvd., Suite 1012
    Los Angeles, CA 90010
    213-731-1166
Provides both technical assistance—screening and testing possible carriers—and support services such as blood banks and summer camps for children with the disease.

Leukemia Society of America
    733 Third Avenue
    New York, NY 10017
    212-573-8484

Cancer

American Cancer Society
    777 Third Avenue
    New York, NY 10017
    212-371-2900

Diabetes

Juvenile Diabetes Foundation International
    60 Madison Avenue
    New York, NY 10010
    212-889-7575
Seeks funds for research and provides support services to juvenile diabetics and their families.

Lupus Erythematosus

The American Lupus Society
23751 Madison Street
Torrance, CA 90505
213-373-1335

National Lupus Erythematosus Foundation
5430 Van Nuys Blvd., Suite 206
Van Nuys, CA 91401
213-885-8787
An organization primarily devoted to researching the causes and cures of lupus.

Multiple Sclerosis

National Multiple Sclerosis Society
205 East Forty-second Street
New York, NY 10017

Skin Diseases

National Psoriasis Foundation
6415 S.W. Canyon Court, Suite 200
Portland, OR 97221
503-297-1545

American Academy of Dermatology
1567 Maple Avenue
Evanston, IL 60201
312-869-3954
The professional society for dermatologists.

United Scleroderma Foundation
P.O. Box 350
Watsonville, CA 95077
408-728-2202
Coordinates information about the disease for the medical profession.

Miscellaneous

Gerontological Society of America
　　1411 K Street, N.W., Suite 300
　　Washington, DC 20005
　　202-393-1411
An organization for professionals of all kinds—from doctors to endocrinologists—interested in the medical state of the aged.

Alternative Medicines

International Academy of Biological Medicine
　　P.O. Box 31313
　　Phoenix, AZ 85046
　　602-992-0589
Another organization of practitioners of traditional and nontraditional medicine. It has a heavy interest in nutrition.

American Holistic Medical Association
　　6932 Little River Turnpike
　　Annandale, VA 22003
　　703-642-5880
A professional organization of physicians experienced in using both allopathic (traditional) and nontraditional therapies such as acupuncture.

Behavioral and Psychosomatic Medicine Societies

American Academy of Behavioral Medicine
　　12890 Hillcrest, Suite 200
　　Dallas, TX 75230
　　214-458-8333
A largely professional organization designed to develop guidelines for applying the principles of behavioral medicine.

Institute for the Advancement of Human Behavior
　　P.O. Box 7226
　　Stanford, CA 94305
　　415-851-8411

Essentially an organization that focuses on offering a program of health care training and in applying concepts such as joining healthy behavior to medical therapy.

Society of Behavioral Medicine
P.O. Box 8530, University Station
Knoxville, TN 37996
615-974-5164

The most important information resource for new developments in behavioral medicine.

Other important information resources for professionals include:

Society for Psychophysiological Research
2380 Lisa Lane
Madison, WI 53711

Academy of Psychosomatic Medicine
70 West Hubbard Street, Suite 202
Chicago, IL 60610
312-644-2623

American Psychosomatic Society
265 Nassau Road
Roosevelt, NY 11575
516-379-0191

American Association of Biofeedback Clinicians
2424 Dempster
Des Plaines, IL 60016
312-827-0440

American Medical Association
535 North Dearborn Street
Chicago, IL 60610

Hypnosis

American Society of Clinical Hypnosis Education and Research Foundation
2250 East Devon Avenue, Suite 336

Des Plaines, IL 60018
312-297-3317

Underwrites workshops to train individuals in the techniques of hypnosis for medical reasons—for pain control in childbirth and dentistry, for example—and in psychotherapy.

International Society for Professional Hypnosis
218 Monroe Street
Boonton, NJ 07005
201-335-4334

A professional society for counselors, doctors, nurses, psychologists, and others who use hypnotherapy.

National Society of Hypnotherapists
P.O. Box 7586
Newark, DE 19711
302-737-8029

Society for Clinical and Experimental Hypnosis
129-A Kings Park Drive
Liverpool, NY 13088
315-652-7299

A professional society that promotes uses of hypnosis in medicine and encourages research into hypnosis.

American Association of Professional Hypnotherapists
P.O. Box 731
McLean, VA 22101
703-448-9623

A professional organization that promotes the use of hypnosis for mental health, controlling bad habits, and aiding the healing process.

American Society of Clinical Hypnosis
2250 East Devon Avenue, Suite 336
Des Plaines, IL 60018
312-297-3317

Sets up training standards and has teaching sessions for professionals interested in using hypnosis.

American Society of Psychosomatic Dentistry and Medicine
4505 Beach 45th Street

Brooklyn, NY 11224
718-266-1188

Promotes the use of hypnosis and acupuncture in dentistry and medicine.

International Imagery Association
P.O. Box 1046
Bronx, NY 10471

This organization promotes imagery research and focuses on the idea of imagery from artistic as well as scientific viewpoints.

Psychotherapy

American Association for Marriage and Family Therapy
1000 Connecticut Avenue, N.W., Suite 407
Washington, DC 20036

A professional society of marriage and family therapists that operates a referral service as well.

American Association for Music Therapy
11 East Forty-third Street, Suite 1601
New York, NY 10017
212-867-4480

Certifies music therapists and promotes the use of music therapy as an adjunct to therapy.

American Association of Religious Therapists
7175 West Forty-fifth Street
Suite 303
Ft. Lauderdale, FL 33314

An organization of psychiatrists, psychologists, and the clergy whose goal is to promote religious perspectives in psychotherapy.

American Dance Therapy Association
2000 Century Plaza, Suite 108
Columbia, MD 21044
301-997-4040

Acts as an information and curriculum center for dance therapists and for schools that wish to include dance therapy in their syllabuses.

American Group Psychotherapy Association
    1995 Broadway, 14th Floor
    New York, NY 10023
    212-787-2618
A professional group that sponsors education and research into psychotherapy.

American Society of Group Psychotherapy and Psychodrama
    116 East Twenty-seventh Street
    New York, NY 10016
    212-725-0046
For those professionals—psychiatrists, psychologists, social workers, and others—interested in using psychodrama as part of their services.

American Psychiatric Association
    1400 K Street, N.W.
    Washington, DC 20005
The professional organization for psychiatrists in the United States.

American Psychological Association
    1200 17th Street, N.W.
    Washington, DC 20036
The professional organization for psychologists.

Association for Advancement of Behavior Therapy
    420 Lexington Avenue
    New York, NY 10170
    212-682-0065

Psychoanalysis

American Psychoanalytic Association
    One East Fifty-seventh Street
    New York, NY 10022
    212-752-0450
Professional group oriented to encouraging the increased use of psychoanalysis in conjunction with other medical specialties.

National Association for the Advancement of Psychoanalysis and the American Boards for Accreditation and Certification
    80 Eighth Avenue, Suite 1210
    New York, NY 10011
    212-741-0515
Operates a training institute and sets the standards for psychoanalytic training.

References Cited

CHAPTER ONE: *The Reunion of Mind and Body*

1. BRUNO KLOPFER, "Psychological Variables in Human Cancer," *Journal of Prospective Techniques* 31 (1957):331–40.
2. YUJIRO IKEMI et al., "Psychosomatic Consideration on Cancer Patients Who Have Made a Narrow Escape From Death," *Dynamic Psychiatry* 8 (1975):77–93.
3. RICHARD A. KIRKPATRICK, "Witchcraft and Lupus Erythematosus," *Journal of the American Medical Association* 245 (1981):1937–38.
4. RENE DUBOS, *Man Adapting* (New Haven: Yale University Press, 1965), 326.
5. LEWIS THOMAS, *The Youngest Science* (New York: Viking Press, 1983), 56–57.
6. FRANZ ALEXANDER, "Psychological Aspects of Medicine," *Psychosomatic Medicine* 1 (1939):17–18.
7. WALTER CANNON, "Stresses and Strains of Homeostasis," *The American Journal of the Medical Sciences* 189 (1935):2.
8. HANS SELYE, *Stress Without Distress* (New York: New American Library, 1974), 14.
9. LAWRENCE LESHAN, "Psychological States as Factors in the Development of Malignant Disease: A Critical Review," *Journal of the National Cancer Institute* 22 (1959):1–18.

10. CAROLINE B. THOMAS, KAREN ROSE DUSYNSKI, and JOHN WHITCOMB SHAFFER, "Family Attitudes in Youth as Potential Predictors of Cancer," *Psychosomatic Medicine* 41 (1979):287–301.
11. GEORGE VAILLANT, *Adaptation to Life* (Boston: Little Brown, 1977).
12. Ibid., 370.
13. THEODORE MELNECHUK, Personal communication.
14. TRUMAN SCHNABEL, "Is Medicine Still An Art?," *The New England Journal of Medicine* 309 (1983):1260.
15. SUSAN SONTAG, *Illness As Metaphor* (New York: Vintage Books, 1979), 3.

CHAPTER TWO: *The Best Defense: The Immune System*

1. FRANZ HALBERG, "Implications of Biological Rhythms for Clinical Practice," *Neuroendocrinology* (Sunderland, Mass.: Sinauer Associates, Inc., 1980).

CHAPTER THREE: *The Brain Connection*

1. TERRY STROM et al., "Cholinergic Augmentation of Lymphocyte-mediated Cytotoxicity: A Study of the Cholinergic Receptor of Cytotoxic T-lymphocytes," *Proceedings of the National Academy of Sciences* 71 (1977):1330–33.
2. ROBERT ADER and NICHOLAS COHEN, "Behaviorally Conditioned Immunosuppression," *Psychosomatic Medicine* 37 (1975):338.
3. MALCOLM ROGERS, "The Influence of the Psyche and the Brain on Immunity and Disease and Susceptibility: A Critical Review," *Psychosomatic Medicine* 41 (1979):159.
4. MARVIN STEIN, "A Biopsychosocial Approach to Immune Function and Medical Disorders," *Psychiatric Clinics of North America* 4 (1981):203–21.
5. HUGO BESEDOVSKY, "Hypothalamic Changes During the Immune Response," *European Journal of Immunology* 7 (1977):232.

CHAPTER FOUR: *Dr. Ishigami's Message*

1. ROBERT ROSE, "Endocrine Responses to Stressful Psychological Events," *Psychiatric Clinics of North America* 3 (1980):251–76.
2. JANICE KIECOLT-GLASER et al., "Psychosocial Modifiers of Immunocompetence in Medical Students," *Psychosomatic Medicine* 46 (1984):7–14.

CHAPTER FIVE: *The Real World Factor*

1. VERNON RILEY, "Psychoneuroendocrine Influences on Immuno-competence and Neoplasia," *Science* 212 (1981):1100–1109.
2. JIM PALMBLAD et al., "Experimentally Induced Stress in Man: Effects on Blood Coagulation and Fibrinolysis," *The Journal of Psychosomatic Research* 21 (1977):87–92.

CHAPTER SIX: *Autoimmunity: The Body Against Itself*

1. RICHARD SURWIT et al., "Diabetes and Behavior: A Paradigm for Health Psychology," *American Psychologist,* March 1983, 255–62.
2. GEORGE SOLOMON and RUDOLPH MOOS, "The Relationship of Personality to the Presence of Rheumatoid Factor in Asymptomatic Relatives with Rheumatoid Arthritis," *Psychosomatic Medicine* 27 (1965):350–60.

CHAPTER SEVEN: *Out of Control*

1. JOHN N. MACKENZIE, "The Production of the So-called 'Rose Cold' by Means of an Artificial Rose," *American Journal of Medical Science* 9 (1886):45–57.
2. JUDITH RABKIN and ELMER STREUNING, "Life Events, Stress, and Illness," *Science* 194 (1976):1013–20.
3. ROGER MEYER and ROBERT HAGGERTY, "Streptoccocal Infections in Families," *Pediatrics,* April 1962, 539–49.

CHAPTER EIGHT: *Cancer and the Mind*

1. RICHARD B. SHEKELLE et al., "Psychological Depression and 17-Year Risk of Death from Cancer," *Psychosomatic Medicine* 43 (1981):117–25.
2. BERNARD FOX, "Premorbid Psychological Factors as Related to Cancer Incidence," *Journal of Behavioral Medicine* 1 (1978):45–134.

CHAPTER NINE: *The Healer Within*

1. THEODORE X. BARBER, "Hypnosis, Suggestions, and Psychosomatic Phenomena: A New Look from the Standpoint of Recent Experimental Studies," *American Journal of Clinical Hypnosis* 21 (1978): 13–27.

Glossary

ACTH (adrenocorticotropin): A hormone trigger secreted by the pituitary gland that acts on the adrenal gland, stimulating the production of corticosteroids.

AIDS (Acquired Immune Deficiency Syndrome): A virus-caused disease that brings about a breakdown in half of the body's immunological defense system. That part of the pattern of immune protection called cell-mediated immunity is severely impaired, leaving the individual vulnerable to a host of bacterial, viral, fungal, and protozoic invasions. The virus is thought to be transmitted through blood and semen.

Adrenaline (*See* Epinephrine)

Adrenal cortex: The outer layer of the adrenals. The cortex is firm and yellowish and comprises the largest part of the gland. Corticosteroids are produced in this layer.

Adrenal Glands: Two glands located adjacent to the kidneys. The adrenal is composed of two portions: an outer part, the cortex, and an inner portion, the medulla. The cortex produces (under control from the pituitary hormone, ACTH) steroid hormones. The medulla produces epinephrine and norepinephrine.

Alexithymia: A condition of human brain and personality development in which an individual is unable to express emotions or feelings in words. Thought to be either the result of an inborn abnormality or a learning disability.

Allergen: A substance capable of inducing allergy or specific hypersensitivity in a susceptible individual.

Allergy: A hypersensitive immune state initiated as the result of exposure to a specific allergen. Characterized by exaggerated reactions to substances, the resulting symptoms are most frequently respiratory, dermatological, or gastrointestinal.

Anaphylactic shock: An unusual and overwhelming allergic reaction in which the body produces a self-administered overdose of histamine in reaction to an antigen after previous sensitization. The result can vary from itching to breathing problems (gasping, wheezing), to total circulatory collapse and heart failure.

Angiogenesis: The process by which the body develops new blood vessels. This is triggered by cancerous body cells to produce a blood supply that feeds nutrients to a tumor and thus speeds up its growth.

Antibody: These are protein chemical compounds produced by the body to combine with specific foreign substances and render them harmless.

Antigen: Any substance that stimulates the immune system to produce an antibody.

Antigenic drift: A very slight change in the structure of an antigen such as a virus. This renders it unrecognizable to an immune system prepared by previous exposure to fight off the virus before the shift occurred.

Anxiety: A state of mind that involves feelings of fear, apprehension, and uncertainty. It often occurs without apparent external stimulus. Anxiety results in physiological changes in the body, the most evident of which are sweating, increased heartbeat, and tremor.

Arsenicoles: Arsenic-rich compounds found in the drinking-water systems of certain areas. These arsenicoles render people who consume them at higher than average risk for skin cancer.

Autoantibodies: An immunoglobulin (antibody) that is formed in response to, and reaction against, a constituent of the tissues of the body that produces it.

Autogenic training: A technique that teaches body relaxation by means of a form of self-hypnosis. Developed about eighty years ago by German psychiatrist Johannes Schultz, the method directs participants to focus their concentration on specific parts of their bodies with verbal messages such as: "my heartbeat is calm and regular." These messages are repeated over and over as in a chant, and then the attention is focused on different part of the body, where the process is repeated.

Autoimmune: Of, relating to, or caused by an immune system that reacts to the presence of an antigen that is part of the body *itself.* The resulting autoimmune disease can be either systemwide or specific to a particular body part. Rheumatoid arthritis and systemic lupus erythematosus are autoimmune diseases.

Autonomic nervous system: The portion of the nervous system concerned with the regulation of the cardiac muscle, smooth muscle tissue, and the glandular system. The autonomic nervous system regulates such things as the rate of heartbeat and digestion.

Bacteria: A classification of microorganisms that are typically unicellular and considered to be plants. They are non–spore forming and live in soil, water, organic matter, and the bodies of plants, animals, and humans. Pathogenic bacteria cause disease in plants and/or animals (including people).

Behavioral medicine: A medical discipline that concerns itself with understanding the role of behavior in the genesis of disease and with helping people to control the state of their own health. It involves therapeutic programs that try to influence and possibly change the behavior and responses of patients. It is multidisciplinary and involves the patient directly in the treatment.

Beta-endorphin: A substance (peptide) produced in the brain and released into the body that has powerful painkilling properties. Beta-endorphin is one of the endorphin groups. Endorphins are found in greatest concentration in the pituitary and are released into the system in reaction to internal or external stress.

Biofeedback: A relaxation technique that uses electronic devices to detect subtle changes in body states by means of sensors. The machines emit signals that inform the patient of the degree of relaxation (or lack of it) achieved by reading changes in brain waves, muscle tension, or electric conductivity of the skin. By learning to use the information from the machines the patient is soon able to reach optimal states of relaxation and even to direct some body functions not normally under conscious control.

Bone marrow: A soft, modified connective tissue consisting of fat cells, maturing blood cells, and numerous blood vessels that fills the cavities of most of the bones of the body. Bone marrow is where stem cells, primitive immune cells, are born.

Brain cortex: The external gray layer of the brain.

Bronchial asthma: A spasmodic contraction of the muscles surrounding the lung's air passageways, resulting in a condition marked by continuous or intermittent labored breathing, accompanied by wheezing, a sense of constriction in the chest, and often coughing and/or gasping. It can be caused by allergy or infection and aggravated by strong emotions.

Cancer: A malignant tumor formed of abnormal body cells that is characterized by the potential for unlimited growth.

Capillaries: Minute, hair-fine vessels that form a network in almost all parts of the body. The capillary walls act as semipermeable membranes for the interchange of various substances and fluids between the blood and tissue fluid. They are the smallest blood vessels in the body.

Carcinogen: A substance or agent that incites or produces cancer. The number of carcinogens in our environment increases yearly as the result of the wastes produced by our technologically advanced societies.

Cartilage: A specialized, translucent fibrous connective tissue found in particular sites of the body such as the joints, nose, and ears. The skeleton of an embryo is made of cartilage and forms the pattern for the bones that develop later as the individual matures.

Catecholamines: A group of compounds, including epinephrine and norepinephrine, that has an action similar to that of impulses conveyed by the sympathetic nervous system.

Cell-mediated immunity: One of two general strategies of the body's immune system. This part of the system is responsible for defense against viruses, abnormal cell growth, and certain intra-cellular parasites. It is the part of the immune system that breaks down in Acquired Immune Deficiency Syndrome (AIDS).

Chronobiology: The scientific study of the rhythm of the body's systems (such as the immunological system). These systems follow distinct patterns of varying efficiency at different times during the twenty-four-hour day.

Control group: A group of subjects (animals or people) involved in an experimental procedure. They are identical in many respects to another group participating in the experiment, except for the absence of the one factor being studied. In the case of experiments made, for example, with new treatments or drugs, the control group is usually given an inactive placebo in place of the experimental substance.

Coping: The pattern or methods—defense mechanisms and reactions—used by individuals to deal with stress, both internal and external. Coping techniques can be learned and altered as the result of certain kinds of psychotherapy.

Corticosteroids: Steroid hormones manufactured by the adrenal cortex. They influence the body's metabolism and protect against stress. These steroids generally suppress immunity.

Cortisol: One of the corticosteroids, it promotes the formation of carbohydrates, is a factor in fat and water metabolism, affects muscle tone and the excitation of nerve tissue, increases gastric secretion, alters connective tissue response to injury, and impedes cartilage production. It is an anti-inflammatory agent.

Cortisone: One of the hormones produced in the adrenal cortex. It is largely inactive in the human body until it is converted to cortisol.

CRF (corticotropin-releasing factor): The hypothalamic hormone that regulates the release of ACTH by the pituitary.

Delayed hypersensitivity reaction: A test for cell-mediated immunity in which a small amount of an antigen is injected into the skin. If the recipient has been previously exposed to the antigen there will be a reaction in the form of a reddened wheal at the site of the injection. It will take two days for the reaction to manifest, as the immune system fights the antigen. No reaction indicates that either the recipient has never been exposed to the antigen or has an impaired immune system. The best-known example is the common skin test for tuberculosis.

Diabetes: Diabetes mellitus is a familial constitutional disorder of carbohydrate metabolism characterized by inadequate secretion or utilization of insulin. Its primary symptoms are excessive amounts of sugar in the blood and urine, thirst, hunger, and loss of weight. One type, insuline-dependent diabetes, is believed to be an autoimmune disease.

Eczema: An inflammatory skin condition characterized by redness, itching, and oozing lesions that become crusted and hardened. It is usually considered to be at least partially psychosomatic, as are many skin ailments.

Endorphin: A substance produced by and released from the brain that acts as a powerful painkiller in the body. The term is derived from *end*ogenous and m*orphin*e. Endorphins also seem to affect learning and memory beneficially and are involved in metabolic and temperature regulation. The amount of endorphins released by the brain is directly related to internal and external stress.

Enkephalin: A natural opiate produced by the brain and other body tissues (*see* **Endorphin**). Part of the body's natural pain-control mechanisms, enkephalins may also play a role in regulation of immune function.

Epinephrine: A catecholamine produced and released by the adrenal medulla in response to stimulation from the nervous system. It is a potent stimulator of the organs regulated by the sympathetic nervous system and may play a role in regulating certain aspects of immune functions. (*Adrenaline* is the British term for epinephrine.)

Estrogen: A generic term for estrus-producing steroid hormones, one of the female sex hormones. Estrogen is used in oral contraceptives, for treatment of the effects of female menopause, and as a palliative in breast and prostate cancer. It may affect the immune system adversely when present in unbalanced levels.

Fungus: Any of a major group of parasitic lower plants that lack chlorophyll. Different types of microscopic fungi can enter the body and cause virulent infections in many different parts and bodily systems, especially when the immune system is suppressed, as in cancer or AIDS.

Genital herpes: An inflammatory skin disease characterized by the formation of small clusters of blisters around the genitals. It is caused by the herpes simplex virus, type II.

Helper T-cells: Thymus-derived lymphocytes, that is, they pass through the thymus or are influenced by it on the way to the tissues of the body. Helper T-cells stimulate antibody production. They are thought to be long-lived and to be responsible for cell-mediated immunity and immunological memory.

Helplessness: An attitude or state of mind in which a person feels powerless and lacking the strength, support, or effectiveness either to cope with specific circumstances or with life in general.

Herpes: A virus-caused skin disease, the symptoms of which are usually clusters of small blisters. The three most common types are herpes simplex, which is usually distinguished by sores around the lips and caused by the type I herpes virus; herpes zoster, or shingles; and genital herpes. (*See* **Genital herpes**)

Heterogenetic: Refers to genetically different individuals, the result of alternation of generations. Outbred rather than inbred. The offspring of animals that are not mated to blood relatives.

Histamine: A substance occurring in the tissues, histamine has three important functions: it causes dilation of the capillaries, which increases capillary permeability and lowers blood pressure; it causes constriction of the bronchial smooth muscle of the lungs; and it causes the induction of increased gastric acid secretion. It plays a major role in allergic reactions. (*See* **Anaphylatic shock**)

Hives: A skin reaction marked by the temporary appearance of smooth, slightly elevated patches that are redder or paler than the surrounding skin and that are usually intensely itchy. Hives can be caused by specific foods, drugs, or emotional stress. Hives is also called *urticaria.*

Holistic medicine: An approach to health whose goal is to treat the entire human being, not just the diseased portion of the patient. While the overall concept of holistic medicine has benefited the science of medicine, some of its attempts to put its theories into action have been antiscientific and potentially dangerous.

Homeostasis: The normal state of the (adult) body in which it is able to maintain a uniform state of health.

Hopelessness: An attitude or state of mind that is despairing, having no expectation of good or success.

Humoral immunity: The immunity acquired after the body is exposed to microbial or other antigens. The role of circulating immunoglobulins (antibodies) is most important in this form of immunity.

Hypertension: An abnormally high blood pressure and the condition that accompanies the high blood pressure, hypertension can be a symptom of a number of disorders or it can be a primary disease entity (essential hypertension).

Hyperthyroidism: Overactivity of the thyroid gland, causing an increase in the basal metabolism and disturbances in the autonomic nervous system. Some types are thought to be psychosomatically involved.

Hypnosis: An verbally induced state of deep relaxation in which attention and concentration are enhanced. The subject is put into a trance by means of visual and verbal suggestions. While under hypnosis, the subject is extremely responsive to suggestions made by the hypnotist and has more than usual access to the unconscious mind.

Hypothalamic-pituitary-adrenocortical axis: That portion of the neuroendocrine system that involves the interaction of the hormones produced by the hypothalamus, the pituitary, and the adrenal glands. It is activated by stress.

Hypothalamus: The portion of the forebrain that forms the floor and part of its side. It has a role in the mechanisms that activate, control, and integrate peripheral autonomic mechanisms, endocrine activity, and many bodily functions (hunger, body temperature).

Imagery: Imagery is a form of therapy based on the use of directed meditation or hypnosis. The subject first achieves a state of relaxation and is then guided by the therapist through an imaginary experience. When used for healing, the mental images may depict the disease cells as villains or dragons or the like, and the immune system cells as powerful "good guys." The principle is to assist the subject to picture in his or her mind an image that, it is thought, will lead to a physical healing.

Immunocompetence: The capacity and ability of the body to produce antibodies and/or to develop cell-mediated immunity after having been exposed to harmful invaders.

Immunoglobulin: Also known as gamma globulin, immunoglobulins form the second major protein of blood plasma. They are subdivided into classes according to their functions. The presence of specific immunoglobulins in the body is a diagnostic indicator.

Immunology: The branch of biomedical science that is involved with the body's response to antigens; the body's ability to recognize "self" and distinguish it from things that are "not self."

Isogenic: The reproduction of animals brought about as the result of mating individuals who are either closely related or who have very similar genetic constitutions. This inbreeding, which produces genetically identical offspring, is usually done to preserve desirable characteristics or to eliminate undesirable ones.

Kaposi's sarcoma: A cancer that is marked by primary symptoms of reddish-purple blotches on the skin, most often on the toes and feet. It is highly malignant. Until the advent of AIDS it was a relatively rare form of cancer; however, it is now seen frequently in AIDS victims.

Learned helplessness: A theory about behavior maintaining that animals and people can be conditioned into a state of extreme helplessness. The individual becomes unable to meet challenging situations with anything other than total capitulation and despair. In both animals and people the result is a state of severe passivity.

Lymph nodes: These are small, rounded bodies that produce lymphocytes to fight invading substances. There are over a hundred lymph nodes distributed throughout the lymphatic system that serve as defense posts for the body against foreign substances causing disease.

Lymphocytes: A white blood cell that is largely produced by lymphoid tissue and participates in humoral and cell-mediated immunity. T-cells are lymphocytes.

Lymphokines: Substances released by lymphocytes that have come in contact with antigens, they are believed to play a role in activating macrophages and cell-mediated immunity.

Macrophages: Macrophages are specialized immune cells that engulf invaders and act as scavengers, thereby cleaning them out of the system. Macrophages play a vital role in alerting the immune system to the presence of antigens, both self- and non-self.

Malignant melanoma: A cancerous tumor consisting of black masses of cells with a distinct tendency to metastasize, or spread rapidly. (*See* **Melanoma**)

Mast cells: A type of white blood cell found in tissue throughout the body that, when stimulated, releases biochemicals such as heparin, an anticoagulant; serotonin, a neurotransmitter; histamine; and other inflammatory mediators.

Meditation: When used in healing, meditation is a technique in which the subject is taught to relax the body completely and to focus the mind in a way that leads to an altered state of consciousness, one that removes the subject from the usual worries and anxieties of daily life. People proficient at meditation can actually bring about changes in their brain waves and other parts of the body's systems not usually under conscious control. It is useful for increasing self-awareness.

Medulla: A general term for the innermost portion of an organ. The adrenal medulla, for example, makes up, with the cortex, the adrenal gland. The catecholamines, epinephrine and norepinephrine, come from the adrenal medulla, as does one of the enkephalins, met-enkephalin.

Melanoma: A tumor comprised of pigmented cells. Not all melanomas are cancerous, but when the term is used alone, it generally refers to a malignant (cancerous) melanoma. (*See* **Malignant melanoma**)

Mesmerism: A form of hypnosis therapy developed in the eighteenth century by Franz Anton Mesmer, a Viennese physician. He healed people by working with what he called "magnetism." This involved elaborate rituals with magnets, hypnosis, and passing his hands therapeutically over the patient's body.

Metastasize: The process by which a disease spreads from one organ or part of the body to another not directly connected with it. With malignant tumors this takes place as a transfer of cancerous cells. All malignant tumors have the capacity to metastasize, though the tendency to spread varies from one tumor to another.

Microbe: A minute living organism, either plant or animal. The term is generally applied to bacteria, protozoa, and fungi that cause disease.

Migraine headache: A vascular headache that involves a complex pattern of symptoms. These include accompanying irritability, nausea, vomiting, diarrhea, or constipation. The duration and intensity of the attack can be quite incapacitating. A tendency to migraines seems to be inherited, but stress and emotional problems are important factors in the frequency and intensity of the attacks.

Mitogen response: A standard immune test that causes certain plant products acting as mitogens to fool immune cells into making new cells by making them "think" they are facing some sort of challenge. It tests the responsiveness of lymphocytes by determining the rate at which mitogen-stimulated cells divide and reproduce.

Monoclonal antibodies: Antibodies produced in the laboratory from a single clone of cells. These tailor-made antibodies are identical to each other and have greatly increased the scope of immunologic research.

Morphine: The principal and most active form of opium. It is highly addictive, but also one of the strongest painkillers ever found. Its use as a painkiller and sedative in the practice of medicine has been largely supplanted by drugs thought to be less addictive.

Multiple Sclerosis: An autoimmune disease in which the nerves of the central nervous system are damaged or destroyed, producing a variety of symptoms such as weakness, lack of coordination, and speech and visual disturbances. The course of the disease is usually prolonged, involving remissions and relapses.

Natural killer cells: Derived from precursor cells in the bone marrow, these null cells specifically seek out and destroy cancer cells and cells infected by viruses. Part of the body's immune surveillance system.

Neocortex: The grey outer layer of the brain and region of higher brain functions.

Neoplasia: The formation of any new and abnormal growth by a progressive multiplication of abnormal cells. Frequently used as a synonym for cancer, although strictly speaking not all neoplasims are malignant.

Neurodermatitis: A skin disease that results in itching but not inflammation. Neurodermatitis is generally brought on by emotional or psychological causes.

Neurohormones: Hormones that either stimulate or are made by the nerves and the nervous system. Well over thirty neurohormones have been identified, and many of them are released into the system as the result of stress. Also called neurohumors.

Neuropeptides: A neurotransmitter made up of amino acids that is active in the brain or nervous system. Endorphins and enkephalins are neuropeptides.

Neurotransmitters: A chemical that is discharged from a nerve-fiber ending to carry messages that bring about direct changes in the body's systems. The neurotransmitter is released by one cell and received by another within a fraction of a second. They are the principal means by which nerves transmit messages from one to another.

Noradrenaline (*See* **Norepinephrine**)

Norepinephrine: A hormone formed naturally in the body's sympathetic nerve endings. The principal neurotransmitter of that system. (*Noradrenaline* is the British term for norepinephrine.)

Null cell: A class of lymphocytes that bears markers for neither T-cells nor B-cells.

Opportunistic infection: An infection, whose cause can be bacterial, viral, fungal, or protozoic, that is capable of adapting to a tissue or host other than its usual one. Tends to occur in immunosuppressed hosts, such as AIDS patients.

Parasympathetic nervous system: One of the two subdivisions of the autonomic nervous system (the other is the sympathetic nervous system). The parasympathetic nervous system slows the body down and aids in digestion, elimination, and relaxation.

Phagocytes: A specialized group of white blood cells that is alert to the presence of invader cells or cellular debris and that circulates throughout the body at all times. When a phagocyte encounters a hostile cell it engulfs, or "eats," it (phagocyte means "cell-eater").

Peptic ulcer: An ulceration of the mucous membrane lining of the esophagus, stomach, or duodenum, caused by an imbalance of acidic gastric juice. Peptic ulcers are considered to be a psychosomatic disorder.

PETT scan: A technique ("positron emission transaxial tomography") that allows nonsurgical study of the brain and heart to observe the biochemical reactions taking place. Using radioactive tagged substances, PETT scanning provides metabolic portraits that reveal the rate at which healthy and abnormal tissues utilize biochemical nutrients. It is a powerful new technique for measuring the metabolic activity of body organs.

Pituitary: A small, oval gland attached to the base of the brain, connected to the hypothalamus by a stalk. Sometimes called the "master gland," the pituitary affects the entire endocrine system through secretion of several hormones.

Placebo: An inert preparation or substance given to a patient (or group of patients within a controlled experiment) in place of a drug or medicinal substance. It can also be a procedure with no known intrinsic value. In either case, the patient is not informed that what is being given or done is not the prescribed medication or treatment.

Plasma: The liquid and colorless portion of the blood in which the corpuscles are suspended.

Plasma cells: A cell of the B-cell lineage that directly secretes large amounts of immunoglobulin.

Pneumocystis pneumonia: An often lethal form of pneumonia that attacks individuals whose immune systems are severely defective. Once considered quite rare in the United States, it is now the leading cause of death among AIDS patients.

Progressive relaxation: A relaxation technique developed in the 1930s by Chicago researcher Edmund Jacobson. It requires that the participant concentrate on and consciously relax different parts of the body in progressive order, i.e., the feet, then the ankles, then the calf muscles, etc.

Prospective study: A study that follows its subjects from the present over a period of time into the future.

Prostaglandin: A hormonelike substance found in tissue throughout the body. There are many types of prostaglandin with varied effects on inflammation and blood vessels. There are large deposits of it in the thymus gland. Research suggests it has a role in the production of T-cells and the regulation of B-cells.

Protozoa: Minute acellular or unicellular animals (microorganisms). Many of them are pathogenic and cause disease in humans and animals. They can be intracellular parasites and thereby cause diseases such as malaria.

Psychoneuroimmunology: The branch of medicine that studies the interrelationships among the mind (psycho), the nervous system (neuro), and the immune system (immunology).

Psychosomatic: Having to do with the relation of the mind (psyche) to the body (soma). Usually, the term is used to refer to diseases that affect the body but have their origins in emotional or psychological disturbances.

Receptors: That part of the surface of cells that recognizes the shapes of molecules. Lymphocytes have receptors for both antigens and neurohormones. Nerve cells only have receptors for neurotransmitters, not antigens.

Relaxation response: A relaxation technique developed by Harvard Medical School cardiologist Herbert Benson that uses many of the traditional forms of meditation—silence, concentration, and passive states of mind—to achieve deep states of relaxation that measurably affect the body's physiology.

Rheumatoid arthritis: A chronic inflammatory disease that mainly affects the connective tissue of the joints. It is the most common autoimmune disease, thought to affect at least 2 percent of the world's population.

Specific etiology: The theory that specific diseases have specific causes was first put forth in the sixteenth century; it had no real influence on the practice of medicine until the discovery of "germs" about 100 years ago.

Spleen: A large glandlike organ located in the upper part of the abdominal cavity near the stomach. It is vital to the immune system and contains phagocytes and red and white blood cells, which it releases into the system as they are needed.

Steroids: Hormones, many of which are produced by the adrenal cortex. The release of some steroids into the system is governed by the release of ACTH from the pituitary. Often used as shorthand for "corticosteroids."

Streptococcus: A strain of parasitic bacteria that takes the shape of a twisted chain. Certain types are extremely pathogenic to humans and animals.

Stress: A vaguely conceived term, usually seen as the response to an outside circumstance or event (stressor), that leads to turmoil and unrest within a person. This disturbance, which is psychological in origin, leads to physiological reactions that then cause distress and may lead to disease.

Stressor: The stimulus (such as working against a deadline) that can lead to a state of stress.

Substance P: One of the neuropeptides, along with endorphins and enkephalins; it carries messages from cell to cell within the immune system. Substance P plays a role in pain regulation and in the regulation of CRF.

Suppressor T-cells: Suppressor T-cells are white blood cells that inhibit the generation or progression of immune responses to specific antigens.

Sympathetic nervous system: The part of the autonomic nervous system that tends to increase blood pressure, increase heartbeat, and inhibit glandular secretions, the sympathetic nervous system prepares the body for fight or flight.

Sympatho-adrenal-medullary axis: A description (by Walter Cannon) of the body's pattern of reaction to *physical* stress that emphasizes the relationship of neurological to hormonal activity.

T-cells: Some of the immune cells that are carried from their origin in the bone marrow to the thymus gland, where they are transformed into T-cells. The "T" in T-cells means "thymus-derived."

Thalamus: The part of the forebrain next to the hypothalamus. It is the relay center for sensory impulses.

Therapeutic touch: A nontraditional therapy developed by Dolores Krieger, professor of nursing at New York University, in which she relieves the pain and distress of illness by passing her hands over the patient. She has formed a method of preparation for the practitioners of therapeutic touch that involves deep meditative states and can be taught systematically.

Thymosin: A class of hormones manufactured by the thymus gland that can affect some immune cells, transforming them into T-cells.

Thymus gland: A pinkish-grey organ about the size of a walnut located just under the breastbone. The thymus is the source of the hormones that regulate the maturation and differentiation of the T-cells.

Thyroid gland: One of the major endocrine glands, it is located in the lower part of the front of the neck, right next to the thymus gland. It secretes thyroid hormones that are involved in regulating the metabolic rate.

Transcendental Meditation: A relaxation technique based on certain forms of Hindu meditation and introduced in the West in the late 1960s. Its practitioners follow a daily discipline of meditation for twenty minutes twice a day.

Trophotropic response: A response of relaxation elicited in animals by means of stimulating the hypothalamus with mild electrical impulses.

Tuberculin: An inactive extract of tuberculosis bacteria used in the Mantoux skin test to determine the presence of tuberculosis in the patient's system.

Tuberculosis: A chronic disease caused in humans and animals by bacteria. It usually affects the lungs in humans, although it can affect any organ of the body.

Ulcerative colitis: Chronic, recurring ulceration of the colon, usually manifested by cramping, rectal bleeding, and loose diarrheal discharges. It often has psychosomatic components.

Vaccine: Dead or weakened pathogenic microorganisms used as an antigen to produce long-term immunity. A crude form of vaccination (against smallpox) was practiced in the Far East centuries ago but did not become a common practice in the West until the nineteenth century.

Vagus nerve: A major nerve of the body that originates in the medulla of the brain and continues through the body into the abdomen. It supplies nerve fibers to the ears, tongue, pharynx, larynx, and other parts of the body.

Virus: A group of minute infectious agents without any independent metabolism. They can only grow and reproduce within living cell hosts, which they do by invading the cell and taking over the machinery and materials of the cell itself.

Warts: Benign skin tumors caused by a viral infection. They seem to be remarkably susceptible to healing by psychological suggestion.

White blood cells: Also called leukocytes, these are the basic immune cells of the body and originate in the bone marrow, liver, and spleen.

Index